Lose weight now!

LOSE WEIGHT NOW !

Introducing the Smart Diet™
Lose weight for real!
Simple. Balanced. Healthy.

ANTONIO MACERATA

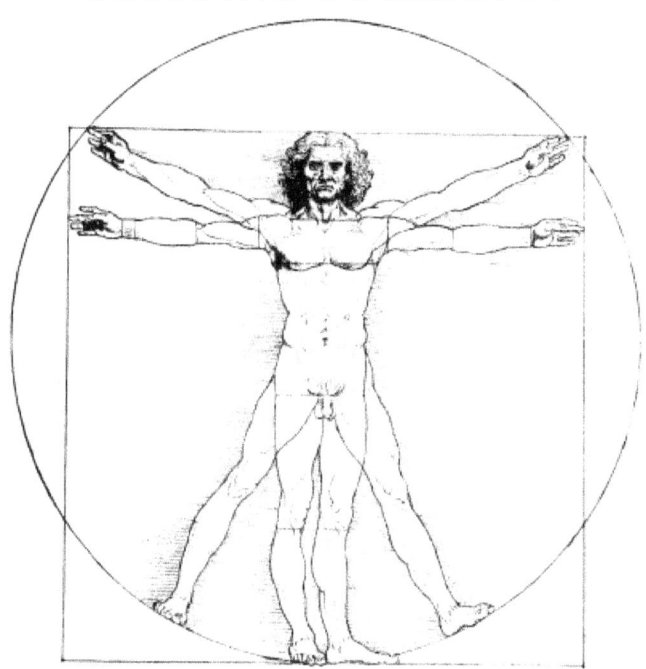

THE BOOK FOR THOSE WANTING TO LOSE WEIGHT IN 2015 AND BEYOND

Lose weight now!

Page left blank intentionally[1,2]

---

[1] There is no reason for this, but it makes the book seem more serious.
[2] But do read the footnotes. Some are useful.

This book is dedicated to my right hand.
You were always there when I felt alone.
You saved my life[3].

---

[3] I play guitar and am right handed. Seriously, what were you thinking?

Lose weight now!

Table of contents

Antonio Macerata

Lose weight now!

Acknowledgments and thanks

This book required a lot of time in research and documentation. Nothing would have been possible without a lot of motivation, dedication and hard work. I therefore absolutely need to start this acknowledgment's section by thanking myself for being so smart, intelligent and so capable of writing such great stuff[4].

More seriously I would like to thank my family and friends (you know who you are and I'm too lazy to mention your names here).

I would like to make a special shout out to four really fun, brilliant young women with bombshell physiques that had the displeasure to work with me at former job (wink)[5].

Since they stressed me with all their questions and thereby led me to get white hair, I have the right to take my revenge. I will do this by embarrassing them in front of the whole world by revealing that:

- The first one would sometimes unintentionally embarrass her former students in front of the whole class when she lost her temper,

- The second one is afraid of spiders and has (from a fashion perspective) a very questionable black leather jacket that she probably could give away for free,

- The third one is afraid of snails,

- The fourth one isn't able to cook "decent" brownies after *at least* two years of trying in vain.

---

[4] If only that were true…
[5] Don't ask me for their emails, they're not single.

Of course, many thanks to you, the Reader, for buying (and hopefully reading[6]) this book. I hope it will help you transform yourself from the "old you" into the "new and improved you" that you want to become.

Peace,

Antonio Macerata

Antonio Macerata
May 30, 2015

---

[6] If you bought it and don't read it, I still get royalties. My win, your loss (lol).

Foreword: Why you should read this book. Or not.

You should definitely **read** this book…

- If you want to lose weight in a durable and healthy way with real results fast,

- If you want to get a better physique through better nutrition and a better lifestyle,

- If you are tired of trying all sorts of diets which don't work for you,

- If you are fed up of hearing all the bullshit marketing and nonsense related to supposedly "effort-free" weight losing methods,

- If you are fed up wasting money on useless "gym" machines, useless dieting books and methods, as well as all sorts of gossip filled magazines with phony advice and silly recommendations,

- IF YOU WOULD LIKE TO TRANSFORM YOUR LIFE BY TRANSFORMING YOUR BODY AND STATE OF MIND.

You should definitely **not read** this book…

- If you are naive and believe that a new "secret" method is going to help you lose weight without effort,

-   If you are credulous and believe that some kind of rare plant used by the ancient Mayas and found in the high mountain chains of Peru will help you lose weight overnight,

-   If you believe that great results come easy without any sweat or tears,

-   If you believe that true love is totally blind and that an "out-of-shape you" will still be able to attract the guy or girl of your dreams,

-   If you accept mediocrity and think that letting your health deteriorate without doing anything is "normal" and "okay" since it's "part of life" and of the aging process,

-   If you are a zombie, vampire or werewolf, because I don't know what are the nutritional requirements and healthy lifestyles recommended for the living dead and other such creatures,

-   IF YOU DON'T HAVE THE COURAGE OR THE WILL TO CHANGE YOUR BODY, STATE OF MIND AND LIFE[7].

Unlike most diet books which have no substance, yet are able to fill hundreds of pages with lots of nonsense and garbage tricks that only work in wonderland and in your dreams, this book has a "straight to your face", real-life factual approach. Therefore it will be short and straight to the point. But do not doubt its effectiveness and its ability to bring you real results fast if you follow the approach suggested.

"Babies are brought to life in blood, sweat and tears by their mothers[8]. Don't expect anything significant in life to come in easy". J. L. Albertson

---

[7] As goes the saying: "Don't try to teach a pig how to sing. It will waste your time and annoy the pig".

[8] This saying only applies to mothers as of course the fathers have the easy part, especially nine months before birth.

Disclaimer: It's all about common sense

I take no responsibility whatsoever, if somebody does stupid things and hurts him/herself after having read or misunderstood the advice of this book.

So if you never did sport in your life, and decide to do 10 hours of cardio exercises to lose weight and then get a heart attack, blame yourself.

If you decide to stop eating sugar because it can lead to fat creation and you end up fainting because of hypoglycemia, blame yourself.

If you want to strengthen your back and decide to go to the gym and squat with a 200kg and then get a spinal disc hernia or bust your knees, blame yourself.

I'll stop it here, but you get the point.

This book was written on the assumption that you, the Reader, are an adult and should behave like one. If you have no common sense and can't think for yourself or take responsibility for your acts, please close this book and watch some junky reality show on TV.

However, if you do understand the facts in this book and follow its advice in a smart way, I warn you, you will be shocked by how much you can improve your body and physique without going through dieting methods which often are just torture for your body and mind.

Of course, if you have a health condition or think you may have one, forget about this book for the time being. Go see your medical doctor to fix/stabilize your condition first.

In life there very are few things that we totally control and that only depend of our own will. Obviously, health is affected by age and genetic predispositions. However, unlike many other things in life such as work or relationships with others, personal fitness and lifestyle choices are largely our own. You cannot blame anyone except your own self for being a lazy couch potato or eating like a pig. No one told you to eat that last pizza or to spend all your afternoons drinking beers and eating barbecues. No one told you not to do sport. It's all your own decisions. It's all in your own hands.

Even with poor genetics and a poor starting place as far as health, you can transform your body in the kind that were sculpted by the ancient Greeks and Romans if you have the courage to change your lifestyle and the determination to stick to these changes. Do it, and you will be handsomely rewarded: not only will you be in better health, you will also have more self-confidence and that will help you in your relationships with others, both professionally, socially and privately.

But choose not to go this route, and at one point in time you will realize that you have gone too far with a long downward slope ahead of you and no way back. One day, your body will tell you "So bitch, you didn't take care of this motherfucker? Now it's payback time. Welcome to the house of pain[9]".

Okay, maybe that's a bit excessive, but in our age and time, our stressful lives, our sedentary lifestyles and the polluted air we breathe just make the odds of living healthy more and more complicated. Without a serious change in lifestyle, we just increase the odds of spending a lot of time ill. We increase the odds of having to depend on other people both physically and financially. It's already a sad thought to think that one may have to spend time in a medical institution for old persons. It's even worse if it's your kids who will have to pay for your healthcare costs or if the money that you could have given to your grandchildren to finance their education ends up paying the cost of your sloppy, "couldn't care less" lifestyle choices.

---

[9] Wow! That sounds dramatic. I should stop watching action movies. :p

You don't want to die with the impression of having stolen part of your kids' and grandchildren's' future and dreams, don't you?

No one will live forever, and many of us will end our lives in a poor physical and mental condition. That's life. But at least we need to ensure that if things go that route, it wasn't because of our decisions. And of course, we need to try to make sure that if that happens, it happens as late as possible.

Ultimately, beyond your genetic health factors, your health is in great part the result of YOUR decisions and YOU will either enjoy the rewards or pay the price. There will be no one to blame in case of failure, but no one to take away the credit from you in case of success!

As said before, it's all in your hands! Don't let people tell you that you are not capable of losing weight! Don't let people make you think that you cannot become a better, healthier person! Do not let people try to keep you down!

Never forget that YOU can become what YOU want to become!

"In life, there are some people who live as spectators watching other people live their lives. I don't want to be like them. I want to be an actor on the stage of life", unknown elite sportsman

"A sound mind in a sound body", ancient Latin quotation

"Too many quotations make me bored", anonymous reader

"Yeah...bro...", anonymous and tired bro

Lose weight now!

Preface or why I am writing this book

The other day[10] I had a lunch with my "Blondie friend" Kim[11,12].

She had invited me to eat at a Lebanese restaurant which is *soooo* good. I was really looking forward to eating a big dish of "chich taouk" with baklava, houmos, etc. Of course, like any "bad boy" I arrived 15 minutes late[13] (if not more). I did not get to eat my houmos because she was in a hurry, but this is besides the point. We started chitchatting and eventually got on the subject of food and dieting. Indeed Kim decided to follow a "caveman diet"[14].

"So what?", you may ask.

Well, you need to understand that Kim is a young woman and that she has a bombshell physique that many women would envy. So Kim going on a diet, moreover an "absurd" diet, is like having an Eskimo from the North Pole worry about what kind of refrigerator he or she should buy.

So I told Kim jokingly that I could easily write two pages to explain her why her diet would not work and what would really work for her[15]. She said "Okay, then write it". I replied "Okay, I'll do it". Challenge accepted. This book is the result of this challenge even though I was not able to limit it to two pages.

---

[10] Actually it was a few months ago.

[11] Of course, this is not her real name, but she will recognize herself.

[12] She may be blondish, but definitely not of the "dumb blonde" kind.

[13] In reality I was in advance, but I was waiting in front of the wrong restaurant. Duh! But it's better for my self-esteem that I write that I was behaving like a "bad boy" rather than admitting I have no sense or orientation whatsoever and that without the map application on my smart phone I would get lost in my very own hometown.

[14] This diet will be explained later in this book.

[15] Considering the fact that she is just fine as she is, she just needs to improve her nutrition habits and continue with her sports.

The book that you hold in your hands (or that you are reading in your e-Book reader) comes from research of no nonsense and factual data. There is no "gossip magazine bullshit" here, no "guru" or "secret tips". Just science and common sense that work in real life. And if I sometimes joke in this book, remember that all the information presented is serious and factual. I just want to keep the book as easy and as fun to read as possible.

I hope you have as much fun reading this book as I did writing it. I hope that you will be able to get the kind of body that you have the motivation to get for yourself. Because even if everyone has his/her own genetic limitations, they are very high and one can really transform one's mind and body into something great!

Introduction: who wants to lose weight?

Every summer, the "people" and "gossip" magazines come out with the same articles on getting back in shape.

Single guys

For men, the articles are often "Get your 6-pack abs ready for summer in 3 weeks" or "How to get back in shape for the beach".

Of course, guys are not naturally interested in their abs or their overall shape. I mean, ask any guy if he doesn't want to drink a beer or have a barbecue? Unless they are under 21 or over 90 years old, none of them will say no. None, except for those who are single.

Indeed, single guys know that an attractive body is necessary if they want to have a small chance of getting laid[16,17]. That's the way the world works. Of course, if you have glasses and are a little bit of an introvert nerd, you're in for a bigger challenge. If on top of that you live in your parents' basement or still ride a bike if you're over 25 years old, then your case becomes so challenging that it makes Frodo's quest to Mordor seem like a health walk on a sunny afternoon. In that case, you will you need much more than a great body and you may have to consider unconventional, desperate measures.

Okay, some guys will just be happy watching free porn on internet, but most single men still preferred getting laid and therefore will look to any diet or "quick fix" to get into shape. As we know, when one is desperate, one becomes naive and credulous. So all of a

---

[16] For shy and skinny guys with no muscles, the chances of getting laid are approximately 0.00000028%. And this only with the condition that they find a girl (or a guy) who is either totally drunk or blind (or both). Same applies for the fat guys.

[17] For all guys over 14, the idea that their girlfriend/boyfriend is a pair of socks is quite depressing. If you're a girl and don't understand the meaning of what I just said, it's normal, it's not for you. Guys know what I'm taking about.

sudden, "people magazines" filled with gossip become as knowledgeable and wise as an encyclopedia or a medical doctor. Of course, in real life these diets and advice don't work and the guys that follow them remain out of shape (and don't get laid).

Married couples

Married couples sometimes don't care too much about their shape since they already have a partner. They often will do the minimum to ensure that their wife/husband/girlfriend/boyfriend doesn't leave them for another (hot) man/woman. However, if the guy stops worrying about his shape, it will often have an impact on his girlfriend/wife/boyfriend/husband who will also stop worrying about the way she/he looks. This will lead to an out-of-shape couple who will prefer dining in restaurants or having drinks *watching* sports rather than *doing* sports. For couples with children, the problem is that being an unfit parent who is unable to do outdoor activities with the kids is very frustrating. This is why even men and women in couple still would like to get in shape.

Women

Women follow a similar pattern to guys, whereby they also want to look attractive, especially in summer when there is less clothing to hide the body's appearance and curves. Women tend to be more self-conscious than guys, and with the body changes related to pregnancies, some become afraid of the aging process, thus prompting them to look for the next new diet, the "one" that supposedly has worked for many Hollywood "stars[18]".

---

[18] Of course, many of the untalented clowns you see in the movies today are nothing close to any kind of real "star". They are totally owned by the likes of Marlon Brandon or Paul Newman. And many of today's female actresses seem like cheap untalented hookers when compared the likes of Audrey Hepburn, Grace Kelly or Marylyn Monroe.

Here too, desperation for results will lead some to become naive and believe all that is written in the magazines. Especially if they are single. That's why articles such as "Boot camp for your booty" or "How to loose your love handles by eating these 10 foods" will become sudden hits. Of course, these diets are "bogus" and "phony" and the only person that benefits from them is their inventor/sponsor who made lots of money in the process.

Bottom line: 99.9% of us want to get (and stay) in good shape

The objectives of this short book are twofold:

1) explain why the popular diets (which you probably know and have followed) just don't work and will not produce the effects you are hoping for

2) explain what diet *really works* in real life over the long haul

I'm writing this short book because I'm *tired* of seeing so much energy being wasted by those seeking for a betting physique in useless diets that in some cases are even *harmful* and *unhealthy*.

I'm writing this short book because I'm *sad* to see that people are led into following "phony" diets that will not help them achieve the results they are seeking and that will leave them frustrated and with less self-esteem than what they had before.

I'm writing this short book because I'm *fed up* at those "gurus" and "specialists" who make tons of money from all these people who are trying to get into shape and who are in a vulnerable state of mind. I despise people who try to take advantage and make money from those that are vulnerable and in need.

That's why this paperback's /e-book's price is so low. I don't want to make tons of money out of it[19]. I just want the most people

---

[19] Of course, if I do make tons of money with this book, I will think about you, dear Reader, while drinking a martini on my yacht surrounded by my many new found girlfriends. Who said that diamonds can't buy love?

possible to read it and find out the facts behind nutrition and a healthy diet. If I really were seeking to make tons of money from a book, I would write a crossover in between recent best-sellers such as "50 shades of Green" and "Hairy Potter"[20].

So I hope you enjoy this book and hope it will help you in your endeavor of getting back into shape. Feel free to share it with all your friends or acquaintances so that some of its wisdom can propagate as fast as STDs in a popular summer beach resort.

Before we get into the heart of this book, let me say just a few more words. This book is not intended to be a medical book or whatever. It's just supposed to be a "real life", no nonsense book on nutrition, how to diet and how to do useful exercise. If you want to lose weight and get yourself a better physique, the one that you really seek to have, you are reading the right book. If you want to learn again how to eat healthy, you are at the right place. If you want to learn what physical activities really are healthy, just continue reading on.

For people wanting to learn more, all the additional information you could need is freely available on the internet. You can also talk with your medical doctor to get more information or to ask your questions. If really you would like to contact me because you have no friends or anyone to bore with questions, you can send me an email at the following address: info@loseweight.ch. You can also check out my web page (www.loseweight.ch).

I will read all emails (which will probably be drowned in junk mail) only every once in a while, but clearly not on a daily basis because I would like to try to get myself a life. So if your question is urgent, ask your medical doctor or check out the internet.

I am not a medical doctor, nor a professional nutritionist, nor an airplane pilot[21]. However, I am interested in living as healthy as

---

[20] It would be a "mommy porn" book with "hot action" taking place in an environment full of wizards and people having magical powers such as looking through the walls of the women's locker room (or the man's locker room) and using magical wands for other purposes than sending magical spells.

[21] I agree with you, this information is quite irrelevant.

possible for as long as possible. In this context I have read quite a bit on nutrition[22] and exercising. I think (subjectively) that I have a good idea of what I'm talking about.

You may have your own opinion and think that I am clueless as far as dieting or exercising because "I ain't got no certification". That's okay with me. You may think that diet XYZ whereby you drink a glass of milk on the night of the full moon is the most effective diet in the galaxy. You may even think that the dieting secrets of Hollywood gurus are useful. That's your opinion, and you can keep it.

But I think that in 2014 everyone should have access to the real facts related to health and nutrition. I don't think that common sense and knowledge are to be reserved to an "elite". So this is my book, and I write what I want. Therefore I get the last word!

Peace,

Antonio Macerata
May 25, 2015

---

[22] There are plenty of information sources on internet. If you don't know where to start, try wikipedia.org.

Lose weight now!

Book structure

The body is like a machine that runs on energy and that requires regular maintenance.

Of course, one could just learn what kind of energy it requires and how to do the maintenance. However we are all different. What will work for someone else may not work for you.

That's why it's important to understand why the body needs certain types of nutrients and what type of maintenance is necessary. That will enable you better to adapt your nutrition and lifestyle to your own body. This will improve the results that you get from your lifestyle choices. In turn, this will increase your motivation to continue on your path of a "better you".

The book is written in a modular way, and you can choose to read one chapter after another or directly pick the chapter that you are most interested in. Of course, reading the chapters in their order is probably better.

The book is structured in 7 parts:

Part 1 (chapters 1-4): in this part I will explain the basics of nutrients (proteins, lipids, carbohydrates, vitamins and minerals) and how they are used in the body.

Part 2 (chapters 5-11): here I will explain the basics of certain human functions (heart, lungs, bones, cartilage, etc) in order to better understand the relationships in between vital biological processes, nutrients and physical exercise.

Part 3 (chapters 12-13): in this part I will focus on how the body loses weight in real-life. No hogwash or baloney here.

Part 4 (chapter 14): this part will focus on some of the well-known diets and show why they don't work in real life despite all the marketing around them.

Part 5 (chapters 15-17): these chapters will focus on what kind of diet really works in real-life. I call it the "Smart Diet"™. I will also explain how to get it started and how to implement it.

Part 6 (chapters 18-21): here I will focus on other health and nutrition topics, including sleep, skincare, libido and erections.

Part 7 (chapter 22): here I will provide further references for those seeking to learn more on proper nutrition and healthy physical exercise.

Chapter 0[23]: Initial assessment of your health

The obvious first step to take before getting in shape is of course to know where you stand as far as health. Not only will this help you measure the progress you have made, but it will also help you determine what could be *healthy* for you as well as what could be *unhealthy* for you. We are all different (luckily!) so understanding the current shape of your body is necessary.

So if you have not done it recently, go get a full health check with your medical doctor. It should include a blood test, a urine test and an ECG (electrocardiogram).

The blood test is important to identify among others:

-   Sugar levels,
-   Iron and other mineral levels,
-   Fat and cholesterol levels,
-   Hormone levels,
-   C-reactive protein levels (indicator of the state of the immune system).

Don't worry! These elements will be discussed in an easy to understand way later in the book. In any case, the results of the blood test will have an impact on the choice of the nutrition plan which is the most appropriate for you.

The ECG test is *very* important to make sure the heart is working properly. The unfortunate thing with heart diseases, heart malfunctionings or just heart weaknesses is that sometimes their symptoms can be very difficult to notice and can be limited to just

---

[23] I'm not too proud on having a chapter 0 in the book, but after all if zero is a number, why does it not deserve to have a chapter of its own? Actually this chapter was written after the others and I was too lazy to renumber them all. I'm really a lazy zero.

fatigue or dizziness. In real life, we see too many children, young adults or adults who die because an undiagnosed heart condition led to a cardiac arrest following too much sport or the consumption of certain stimulants. So really, get an ECG. It's a routine check. It's done quickly and is not painful at all.

Also discuss with your doctor the state of your articulations, back, neck, etc, as you need to understand if you have any medical conditions which could limit your ability to do certain physical exercises.

I'm not going to keep it secret any longer: trying to lose weight only through dieting but without doing any kind of physical exercise is like trying to teach a pig how to sing. It just won't work, no matter how hard you try. If you do think that a proper nutrition without any physical exercise can get you the physique that you want, please continue reading this book so I can show you how wrong you are (or prove me that you are able to teach a pig how to sing)[24].

Once the medical checks have been done and before you really get into the process of building the physique of the "new you", take some pictures of yourself in underwear (the "old you"). And then, every two weeks, repeat the same thing and take new pictures[25]. Indeed if you look at yourself everyday in the mirror, it's difficult to notice changes in your body. However other people will notice the changes, and if you look at the pictures side by side, you too will notice the changes and you will be even more motivated in continuing your journey to get (and maintain) the physique and health that you want.

Lastly, take your weight, your waist and hip measurements. You will then take again these metrics at least on a monthly to measure the progress you make.

---

[24] As far as getting into shape, 70% is nutrition and 30% is physical exercise.
[25] If you're a hot chick, please feel free to share some pictures with me. ^_^

Part 1: Understanding the basics of nutrition

Before we get into the myths of popular diets, you should understand the basics of nutrition and the role different nutrients play in your health.

Basically the food we eat can be broken down into four categories whose function and importance I will describe hereafter. Don't worry, I'm not going to try to bore you to death with biological/medical terms. For that, you can go on the internet. I'll keep my stuff as easy to understand as possible using plain and simple English.

The four categories of nutrients we eat are as follows:

- Proteins,
- Lipids,
- Carbohydrates,
- Vitamins and minerals.

That's it. You see, it's easy. Now let's dig a little deeper into these nutrients.

Lose weight now!

Chapter 1: Proteins

People often think of proteins as the stuff that goes into the muscles and that only bodybuilders need. But there is *much* more to that story.

There are approximately 20 amino acids (which are the building blocks of protein), 9 of which are considered essential because the body cannot make them, which means that they must be supplied by our diet. The five main functions of protein are listed below.

1.1. Building and repairing tissue

Protein is essential to grow, build and repair human tissues. If goes way beyond muscle tissue.

1.2. Making chemical reactions happen

One of the biggest uses of proteins in the human cells is enzymes, which catalyze chemical reactions. In plain English, enzymes are molecules which are necessary to make chemical reactions happen (without them nothing happens). Enzymes are catalysts. As example, enzymes are used in the processes of DNA manipulation, such as DNA replication or DNA repair. No cell could repair itself or multiply if there were not enough protein in the body.

1.3. Transmitting signals

Proteins also are used as a way to transmit a signal from certain cells in the body to others located far away. Insulin, for example, is a protein that helps the body regulate the sugar levels in the blood. Antibodies are also proteins and are vital in the immune system.

1.3.1. A few words on simple on C - reactive protein

I think it is important that you know what is the C - reactive protein (known as CRP) since it's one of the key elements that are analyzed by doctors when looking at a blood test. So here are a few words about it.

This protein is found in the blood and its levels rise in the response to inflammations within the body. CRP is therefore an indicator of the state of the immune system and thus a symptom of problems within the body.

The CRP is made in the liver[26] and apart liver failure, there are few known factors that interfere with CRP production. The levels of CRP in the blood will increase if there are bacterial, viral, fungal or other inflammatory diseases. The way CRP works is that it will bind to the surface of the dead or dying cell thus "identifying" it so it can be eaten (phagocytosed) by the macrophages (white cells). CRP thus participates in the clearance of infected, dead or dying cells. Of course, once the source of the inflammation has been eliminated and that all infected, dead or dying cells have been removed, there is no further need to "mark" cells and the CRP levels will go down.

1.4. Carrying useful molecules

Proteins also are used as "carrier molecules" which means that they help carry certain molecules from one part of the body to another. The most "famous" example is hemoglobin which transports oxygen in the body.

---

[26] This is another reason why to take care of the liver. Foods/substances that are good for the liver and those that are bad for the liver will be discussed later in this book.

1.5. Conferring stiffness[27]

Proteins also confer stiffness and rigidity to otherwise fluid tissues. For example collagen is the protein which keeps the skin "elastic" and helps it keep its "volume". If skin is exposed to too much sun (ultraviolet), or with the aging process, the collagen will start to deteriorate which leads to a thinner, weaker skin where wrinkles will start showing up. The spinal discs are also composed of material similar to collagen. Collagen is also a critical component of bones and of the placenta.

Keratin is found in hard or filamentous structures such as hair and nails.

You got it, no healthy back without protein. No pretty hair or skin without protein. So ladies, please stop saying you don't need protein because you don't do a lot of sport or don't want muscles!

---

[27] I'm talking about cellular stiffness. If you're a guy and thinking about your "other stiffness", you are definitely not reading the right book.

Chapter 2: Lipids

Lipids are basically the "fats" that people talk about. However, contrary to what some may think, fats are essential to any form of life. There are also several types of lipids, so let's try to understand some of their purposes and see what is good and what is bad for our health. This is not a chemistry book, so I will limit the chemical notions to a minimum. What matters is that you understand the bottom line.

2.1. Fatty acids

Fatty acids are non-water soluble molecules. These molecules are vital in the frame of many biological processes. For example, thromboxane is used in the process of clot formation (thrombosis) without which we would bleed to death if we cut ourselves. Another example is docosahexaenoic acid (DHA) which is an omega-3 fatty acid that is a primary structural component of the human brain's cerebral cortex, sperm, testicles and retina.

Fatty acids can be called "saturated" or "unsaturated". Saturated means that they are saturated with hydrogen atoms. Unsaturated fats have less hydrogen atoms as there are more "carbon-carbon" chemical links and less "carbon-hydrogen" links.

Description of fatty acids

Fatty acids are long molecules with chains of carbon and hydrogen atoms. Without getting too deep into chemistry, what is important to understand is the following:

1. When broken down, fatty acids release a lot of energy at molecular level (ATP). Therefore fatty acids are key to store and release energy in the body.

2. Fatty acids are key molecules for life and have much more importance than just being a source of energy. Fatty acids can be found in many tissues and areas of the human cells.

3. There are two big categories of fatty acids: unsaturated fatty acids (also called unsaturated fats) and saturated fatty acids (also called saturated fats).

Classification of fatty acids	
Unsaturated fats	**Saturated fats**
1. Unsaturated fats have one or more double carbon-carbon bonds. 2. Unsaturated fats (with the exception of transfats) are considered more healthy than saturated fats as they tend to increase the production of "good cholesterol" and limit the production of "bad cholesterol" (see section 2.2.1 below). 3. Unsaturated compounds are more likely to be liquid but more importantly, they are more likely to oxidize than saturated fats. This is an important health point so I will discuss it below in section 2.1.1.	1. Saturated fats only include single carbon-carbon bonds and therefore contain a high number of hydrogen atoms. 2. Generally saturated fats release more energy (calories) than unsaturated fats, but this is not really important. 3. Often saturated fats tend to favor the production of enzymes which increase insulin resistance (i.e. they reduce the body's ability to remove sugar from the blood, thus leading to diabetes and cardiovascular problems). 4. High levels of saturated fat intakes are linked to other diseases than cardio-vascular. They are linked to several types of cancer (breast cancer, colorectal cancer, ovarian cancer, prostate cancer, etc).

4. Unsaturated fats can be classified in several categories:

   1. Mono-unsaturated fats

   2. Poly-unsaturated fats

   3. Transfats

   4. Omega fatty acids

   The different categories of unsaturated fatty acids will be described in the table in the next page.

5. High intakes of saturated fats are also linked to bone demineralization and higher risks of osteoporosis.

6. Saturated fats have a higher melting temperature than unsaturated fats and generally stay solid at room temperature. This is why the food industry tends to put a lot of saturated fats in foods.

7. Not all saturated fats are bad! Some (rare) saturated fats are vital in many functions including in the immune system and transport of minerals to certain tissues.

Classification of unsaturated fatty acids	
Mono-unsaturated fatty acids (MUFA)	There is only one double carbon bond (C=C). All the rest are simple carbon bonds. MUFA's tend to increase cell membrane fluidity but are very sensitive to oxidation (see 2.1.1. below). Furthermore they can increase insulin resistance.
Poly-unsaturated fatty acids (PUFA)	PUFA's have several double carbon bonds (C=C). PUFA's include DHA, Omega-3 and other very useful molecules to reduce cardiovascular diseases as well as to promote overall health. Omega fatty acids will be discussed in section 2.1.3 below.
Transfats	Unlike the other unsaturated fatty acids, transfats increase the "bad cholesterol" and decrease the "good cholesterol" (see section 2.1.2 below). The chemical processes are complex and are beyond the scope of this book. They will therefore not be explained.

2.1.1. A few words on oxygen, oxidation and free radicals

Oxygen is vital to life. However, few people realize that oxygen is a highly toxic molecule and is the chemical agent that is the cause of aging and ultimately death in all living things. In clear, from a chemical point of view, the oxygen atoms are the main cause of the aging process.

Without getting into Nobel Prize level chemistry, this is how it works.

Oxygen is of course plentiful in the body. As humans we breathe it. It's also all around us and plentiful on earth. Oxygen is found in the air where it makes up 21% of the atmosphere. In its gas form, oxygen is known as dioxygen and comprises two oxygen atoms (chemically written O^2).

Oxygen found in the O^2 form will not react easily react with other atoms. However in the presence of hydrogen (found in water among others), there can be a chain of chemical reactions that can lead to a series of electrically charged molecules containing oxygen. These electrically charged molecules are referred to as "ions" or "free radicals".

These ions/free radicals are *electrically unstable* and will *react quickly* with other atoms/molecules. In the case of the oxygen derived ions, these ions will degrade many vital molecules, including the DNA, protein molecules, as well as many cellular structures including the mitochondria. Basically all molecules with carbon-carbon bonds (double carbon bonds) can be degraded by oxygen derived ions.

By degrading, I mean that the molecules "attacked" by the oxygen ions will be altered and will no longer be able to fill their initial purpose. Worse, they may even become dangerous due to changes in their atomic composition, electrical charge or electrical properties.

Over time, free radicals accumulate and degrade more and more molecules, thus not allowing the body to heal or repair itself. For exmaple, the oxygen ions which "attack" the DNA molecules will lead to "DNA errors" which will be replicated when the cells multiply.

While most of the errors in the DNA are corrected after the cell replication (or that the dysfunctional cell is killed), over time the amount of "errors" in the DNA will accumulate. These errors will eventually lead the body to be less and less functional. Skin becomes less elastic, the immune system becomes less effective, bones become less dense and even the neural system can eventually decay.

Oxygen is therefore a necessary atom for life, but it's also the single biggest factor that drives the aging process.

One of the best known illnesses related to the oxidation process is cancer whereby healthy DNAs of cells are damaged. Since free radicals can damage so many key molecules within the cell, the human body has ways to limit the action of free radicals.

Antioxidants are molecules that inhibit the oxidation of other molecules. Flavins[28], enzymes and other types of molecules also play this role. In addition the body also has its own repair mechanisms. Remember that every day, *each* cell can have anywhere in between one thousand and one million molecular lesions[29].

However oxidation is a natural process within the body and it cannot be avoided, stopped or reversed. It's part of life. The objective for us is to try to have this process go as slowly as possible. Our nutrition and lifestyle is an important part of this. In chapter 21, I will mention some of the foods/drinks which contain high levels of antioxidants. In addition regular physical exercise has been found to increase the antioxidant mechanisms of the body.

2.1.2. A few words on transfats

Transfats are another much publicized type of molecules. As said above, transfats are an unsaturated fatty acid molecule which contains one or several carbon-carbon bonds. Transfats can be of animal or vegetable origin and can be found in meat, milk or oils.

The food industry sometimes uses a process called "hydrogenation" which ads hydrogen molecules with the objective to increase the saturation levels of the fats used. The food industry continues to use

---

[28] This will be discussed later in chapter 21.
[29] In the case the cell cannot be fixed, it will go through the process of apoptosis (programmed cell death). In a healthy adult, in between 50 billion and 70 billion cells die on a daily basis through this process. Since the human body has around 10 trillion cells, programmed cell death represents approx. 0.7% of the total cell count.

partially hydrogenated transfats for several reasons: 1) these molecules increase the shelf life of the products and therefore decrease the refrigeration requirements, 2) transfats can suspend solids at room temperature (thus enabling some foods to look good at room temperature) and 3) transfats are cheaper than other oils.

Bottom line: transfats are cheaper, that's why the food industry uses them. However they will affect your health, even those that are partially hydrogenated. Indeed, transfats increase significantly the risk of heart disease as they increase the proportion of "bad cholesterol". This is discussed below in sections 2.2.1 and 2.2.2.

Transfats also tend to increase the risk of other medical conditions such as Alzheimer, diabetes, cancer, infertility in women, depression, liver conditions, etc.

2.1.3. A few words on omega fatty acids

There are three groups of omega fatty acids:

Omega 3: these molecules are essentially found in fish oils. Their intake has been linked to a reduction in cancer and heart issues. They are also anti-inflammatory and can help against certain conditions such as arthritis or Crohn disease. They also help reduce the neural aging process (dementia) and help in certain psychiatric conditions (bipolar conditions or depression). During pregnancy, the intake of Omega 3 fatty acids is critical to the good development of the neural cells (brain) of the fetus.

Omega 3s are called this way as the double carbon bond occurs in the 3rd position counting from end of the molecule.

Omega 6: these molecules are often found in vegetable oils. Excessive omega 6 intake as compared to the intake of omega 3 can lead to increased risk of inflammatory diseases or cancers. Research suggests that it's the combination of omega 6 with air pollution, cigarette smoke or second hand smoke that triggers the inflammatory issues.

Omega 6 are found in all vegetable oils, many cereals, nuts, etc.

Omega 6s are called this way as the double carbon bond occurs in the 6th position counting from the end of the molecule.

Omega 9: these molecules are not essential fatty acids, as the body can create them from omega 6 molecules. This is unlike the omega 3 and omega 6 molecules that the body is not able to synthesize on its own. Omega 9 molecules are found in many of the tissues of the body (cartilage, adipose tissue, etc). Some omega 9 fatty acids also serve in critical parts of the nervous systems such as the myelin[30] of nerve cells.

2.2. Glycerolipids and the issue of cholesterol

Glycerolipids are the "fat" that we all know and that are the molecules that store energy for future uses. When metabolized, they yield large quantities of adenosine triphosphate (or ATP) which is the molecule which is the source of cellular energy.

The most "known" type of "fat" are the triglycerides which can be saturated or unsaturated (same as for the fatty acids).

2.2.1. A few words on cholesterol

I think it is important that you better understand cholesterol because here too, the media comes up with many contradictions. Often what is heard can be confusing or even misleading.

Cholesterol is a chemical molecule which is classified in the category of "fats". Cholesterol is a necessary and vital structural component of mammalian cell membranes. It is required to establish proper membrane permeability and fluidity, i.e. the exchanges in between a living cell and its environment. Remember, a cell is like a household, it lives in the frame of an environment. Therefore it

---

[30] This is the electrically insulating layer around the axons of the nerve cells. Multiple sclerosis is one of the many conditions which can occur if this layer degenerates.

needs to get stuff from the "outside" (e.g. energy, and the other necessary molecules for its functioning) and get some stuff "outside" (e.g. waste, or the "things" that the cell produces and that is needs to give to other cells). Without their permeable membranes, cells would not be able to live.

One can therefore easily understand the importance of the cell membranes of which cholesterol is a key component. Bottom line, if you have no cholesterol, you are probably not reading this book as you would not be alive.

Cholesterol is also a building block in the production of bile (which helps absorb certain vitamins and certain molecules). Cholesterol is also a building block in hormones such as testosterone and estrogens. In fact, cholesterol is necessary to produce many hormones. As said in the introduction, this isn't a medical book so I'm not going to list them all. If you want to get the list, go on internet. In any case, I hope you see why cholesterol is vital for the human body.

Cholesterol is not soluble in water. Therefore it has to be transported in the circulatory system by "carrier" molecules which are called lipoproteins. There are five categories of lipoproteins which are classified according to their density, but in the media we usually hear about low-density lipoprotein (LDL) which is also called "bad cholesterol" and high-density lipoprotein (HDL) also known as "good cholesterol".

LDL molecules can very in size and density but they have a molecular structure whereby their smaller size makes them easier to penetrate the interior of the walls (endothelium) of the blood vessels. On the other side, HDL molecules are "bigger" and thus less susceptible to go through the walls of the blood arteries. To take an image, its like if you have a sieve (or filter) and the LDL molecules are small and go through the sieve (or filter), while HDL molecules are too big and don't go through.

This is important as if LDL molecules go through the walls of the blood vessel, they will create an immune reaction where macrophages (the cells that "eat" the intruders in the frame of the immune system) are going to phagocyte (i.e. "absorb") them. Indeed, the immune system "knows" that LDL molecules are supposed to stay in the blood stream and that they are not supposed to go trough the blood vessel's wall (i.e. endothelium).

The chemical residue of the decay of the macrophage and the LDL molecule is the "plaque" which is the basis for atherosclerosis, i.e. the clogging of the arteries which can lead to death through the clogging of the heart arteries (heart attack) or those of the brain (cerebral vascular accident). LDL also tends to oxidize faster, thus increasing anti-inflammatory and immune reactions which can also lead to plague formation.

I will talk later in the book about nutrition and what foods to avoid/favor to try to decrease LDL and increase HDL levels. In any case, the more "fat" (or triglycerides) one eats, the more cholesterol will end up in the circulatory system. The proportion of HDL and LDL is partly genetic and partly related to nutrition. Some molecules such as phytosterols help reduce LDL levels. Phytosterols can be found in certain foods, but as said before, I will talk about this further in the book.

We know that certain foods and certain medicines can help reduce the LDL molecules in the blood stream and/or increase HDL molecules in the blood stream, thus reducing future risks of plaque formation in the blood vessels.

However there is no effective medicine that can help remove the *existing* plaque from the blood vessels. This is why *prevention* of high LDL levels is so important. Once the damage is done, it's not possible to repair it based on today's medicine. I.e. at the time of my writing, there is no known way to "unclog" the arteries that are damaged. A healthy lifestyle can reduce future atherosclerosis, but cannot do anything to "fix" the "clogging" that has *already* occurred and that is *permanent.*

There are recommended maximum levels of triglycerides and LDL in the blood, as well as minimum recommended levels of HDL. The following levels are considered "normal".

- Triglycerids: < 2.0
- Total cholesterol: < 5.0
- HDL cholesterol: > 1.0
- LDL cholesterol: < 3.0
- Ratio total cholesterol/HDL: < 5.0

Units are expressed in millimoles[31] per liter (mmol/l).

2.2.2. Atherosclerosis, HDL genetic profile, statins

Since atherosclerosis and cholesterol is such an important health risk, I would like to go touch some important points.

1) Each person has a different and unique genetic profile. This holds true for cholesterol and each person will have his/her own cholesterol profile. I.e. certain people are born with "good" genetics, i.e. a high natural proportion of HDL vs. LDL. Other people will have a "poor" cholesterol profile whereby LDL production is much higher. That's life.

2) Like oxidation (see point 2.1.1. above), atherosclerosis is a "natural" process that starts in the early teens in kids and that continues throughout life. Obviously since we all have LDL molecules, we all eventually have some of them going through the endothelium where they will lead to plaque formation. So don't get panicked because of it. It's part of life. Death too is part of life and needs to be accepted. The point is that this ultimate fate can be *significantly deferred* in time because there is no urgency for death or heart diseases. This is why good eating habits and healthy lifestyles are so important.

---

[31] Without getting into chemical stuff, you just need to know that millimoles measure the number of "units" of the measured "substance" per liter of blood.

3) There is a class of medical drugs called statins. Statins help decrease LDL cholesterol levels and are prescribed by medical doctors for people (usually 45 and older) who have serious cholesterol issues. These medical drugs have become really popular, and some of their names have even become household names (Lipitor, Crestor, Zocor, etc)[32]. Statin sales around the world are well beyond USD 30bn per year! So it's a big business and reflects a big health risk in the population due to poor eating habits and unhealthy lifestyles.

As said before, statins cannot do anything against the plaque that is already in the arteries which is why prevention is important. However statins do decrease LDL levels and they also reduce the inflammatory response if the LDL goes through the walls (endothelium) of the blood vessel.

4) The good news is that one can increase naturally the proportion of HDL cholesterol by the following:

- Regular physical activity ("cardio")

  Regular exercise will increase the proportion of HDL cholesterol vs. LDL cholesterol. The reasons are quite complex and will not be discussed here. But when the body is under physical "stress", changes in metabolism will favor the production of HDL as the body needs to increase the speed/efficiency of certain chemical reactions to ensure that all the cells involved in the physical activity (even if they are in "support functions") are able to continue to function properly. This is why the body will produce more HDL cholesterol.

---

[32] Full disclosure: I didn't get paid by any of these pharmaceutical companies to put up these names here.

- Reducing the levels of triglycerides and transfats in the blood

This is done through a better nutrition and quality of the fats eaten (i.e. significantly reduce the intake of saturated fats).

- Stop smoking

Some of the chemicals found in cigarette smoke (such as acrolein) will trigger a change in the process of the production of lippo-proteins which will decrease HDL cholesterol and therefore increase LDL cholesterol. Again, I will not get into the detailed chemical reactions that lead to this, but you get the point.

Chemicals in smoke will also tend to increase the inflammatory response when LDL cholesterol goes through the endothelium. In short, there will be more white cells that will go the problem area. This will increase the plague formation.

2.2.3. A more in-depth look at atherosclerosis

In chapter 5 (section 5.5), I will revisit the process of atherosclerosis, including the issues of body inflammatory response to nutrients. Atherosclerosis is a very important issue but before we get into more details on this subject, we need to discuss some other points.

2.3. The other lipids

Cool! If you are reading these lines, it's that you have survived the pretty geeky section on cholesterol and did not fall asleep. However I sense some fatigue on your side, so I'll wrap up the lipids section by saying that there are many other types of lipids which are used in a variety of biological processes.

Glycerophospholipids are used in the frame of cell signaling (i.e. the way cells send and receive signals from other cells). The human brain contains a lot of glycerophospholipids and any alteration in their composition can lead to neurological disorders.

Other lipids also absorb, store and metabolize vitamins but I will not get into more detail.

2.4. Short conclusion on lipids

As you can see, the issues around lipids are much more complex than the simplistic view of "fats are bad". What you should take from this chapter is the following:

1. Most fats (saturated and unsaturated) have an essential role in human life.

2. Unsaturated fats should be taken in much greater quantity than saturated fats (generally the ratio should be >3:1).

3. Omega 3's should be taken in greater quantity than omega 6's (ratio >1:1).

4. The intake of transfats should be minimized.

5. The intake of fats should be balanced with the other nutrients.

6. Antioxidants are an important part of nutrition.

7. Regular exercise is essential to control fat accumulation in the body (including in the arteries).

8. If you smoke regularly and don't want to stop, you might as well forget about dieting or eating healthy because you are going to accumulate so many problems that being overweight will probably be the smallest of your concerns if you end in hospital.

Chapter 3: Carbohydrates

Carbohydrates are often referred to as "sugars" and considered "bad". As you will see, this is a highly inaccurate and simplistic statement.

3.1. Carbohydrates as energy source

A carbohydrate is an organic compound that consists only of carbon, hydrogen, and oxygen[33]. In chemistry these molecules are referred to as saccharides. Contrary to proteins or lipids which are building blocks for other molecules, carbohydrates are not used to produce other molecules.

Carbohydrates (hereafter "carbs" because I'm getting lazy typing) are used as a source of energy for the human body. In theory, one could think that carbs are not necessary and that the body could just burn lipids (fats) or proteins to generate energy. This is not true.

First, the neurons (brain cells) cannot burn fat for energy. They need glucose (the simplest form of sugar). Second, transforming lipids into energy (glucose) is a long process which takes some time. Therefore if the body needs energy quickly, the conversion of lipids into glucose is not going to deliver the energy on time. It would be like being delivered food tomorrow when you are hungry today. It's just too late. That's why the body needs, and stores carbs. Third, not all proteins can be used as source to generate energy.

When looking at energy produced (measured in calories per gram), things look as follows:

---

[33] An interesting fact is that all atoms, except hydrogen are created in the frame of fusion processes within the cores of stars and during star supernovae. Therefore we are all indeed "star dust".

- Lipids: 9 kcal/g,
- Proteins 4 kcal/g,
- Carbs: 4 kcal/g.

So yeah, lipids produce the most energy (as measured in kcal) per gram consumed, but we have seen before that a) they cannot produce energy quickly if the body needs energy *now* and b) they can have very negative health consequences (high LDL and triglyceride levels in the blood). Proteins cannot be converted quickly into energy either. Furthermore, as said before, not all proteins can be used to produce energy. Bottom line: carbs are *necessary*.

Carbs are divided into four groups depending on the length of the molecular chain: monosaccharides, disaccharides, oligosaccharides, and polysaccharides. Think of carbohydrate molecules like chains made out of building blocks. While the building blocks are the same, one can have either very short chains (or even a chain of only one building block) or a very long chain containing many building blocks.

The shorter chains are usually referred to as "sugar" in every day's language. In nutrition vocabulary they are referred to as "simple sugars" or "simple carbs". For example glucose and fructose are two small molecules (or chains) and thus can be converted almost immediately into energy which is why they are found in all the energy sport drinks. It's because sugars can be converted so quickly into energy that we have some sugar in the circulatory system.

The longer chains of carbs (also referred to as complex sugars) are broken down into smaller chains that can be absorbed by the body and transformed into glycogen. Glycogen is stored in the liver cells and in the muscle cells as a reserve in case immediate energy is needed.

The body will go through the following process when it needs energy. The steps go in the following, invariable order:

1) First, use the sugar which circulates in the blood stream (blood sugar).

2) If this is not enough, use the glycogen from the liver and the muscle cells to generate energy.

3) If this is not enough, use the lipids (fats) and convert them into energy.

4) If this is not enough, use the proteins from muscles to transform them into energy.

In a blood test, the normal fasting glucose levels should be in between 3.9 and 6.1 mmol/l. Below this range there is a condition of hypoglycemia and above a condition of hyperglycemia. Hyperglycemia will be discussed below so I will discuss shortly hypoglycemia. This condition can lead to fatigue, dizziness, attention disorders and fatigue as basically the brain doesn't have enough energy. If hypoglycemia becomes a more persistent state, it can lead to severe medical problems such as tachycardia, seizures, sight problems as well as nervous problems including amnesia or delirium.

In most cases temporary hypoglycemia can be treated by the ingestion of simple carbs (sugars).

3.1.1. A few words on simple vs. complex carbs and diabetes

Since type II diabetes is one of the fast growing diseases in the world, it is important to understand how it's related to carbs. I will not get into type I diabetes which is a condition which is unrelated to nutrition but comes at birth. On the other hand, type II diabetes can be avoided through healthy nutrition.

Complex carbs, those with the longer chains, take more time for the body to be absorbed since the chains need more time to be broken. Since most of the time the body needs a steady source of energy over a long period of time, complex carbs are a very efficient energy source as they are *progressively* released into the blood.

This contrasts with simple carbs who end up very quickly in the blood, all at the same time. Everybody knows about hypoglycemia which is when people don't have enough sugar in their blood and either feel tired or even pass out. However people don't realize that there is also an upper limit of how much sugar the blood can have. Too much sugar in the blood for long periods (hyperglycemia) is a serious condition which can cause many long-term health problems including heart diseases, eye, kidney, and nerve damage.

Since the body cannot work with high levels of sugar in the blood, it will use insulin (produced by the pancreas) as a signal to tell the cells to start absorbing more sugar in order to get some of the excess sugar out of the blood stream. Basically insulin has, among others, the following functions: 1) it enhances entry of glucose into cells; 2) it enhances storage of glucose as glycogen, or the conversion of glucose into to fatty acids (and then fat).

So what's the problem with eating lots of simple carbs since the body has mechanisms to deal with higher sugar levels? Well there are many problems:

1) As said before, high levels of blood sugar over a long period of time can lead to serious diseases.

2) When the body "panics" because of high glucose levels, it will basically rush the production of glucose into fat (and we have talked in the section about lipids what high levels of lipids can lead to as far as atherosclerosis, etc).

3) The pancreas cells which produce insulin can basically do "burnouts", i.e. either they stop working at all or they only work a little bit. This is *irreversible* and becomes a *permanent* condition. No medicine can help "burned out" pancreas cells produce again insulin.

In plain English, once the pancreatic cells are fucked up, they're fucked up for good. So at this stage, one has type II diabetes and injections of insulin become necessary. This is why prevention is necessary.

Diabetes type II, while not life threatening if one does the daily injections, remains a very serious disease which is chronic (i.e. cannot be cured) and which increases the risk and complications related to other diseases. For example, diabetes increases the risk of cardiovascular diseases by a factor of 2 to 4 (!), it increases the risk of blindness and kidney failure. It has also been associated with an increased risk of cognitive dysfunctions such as Alzheimer's disease.

I don't want to go into more in detail on this subject, but I will end up by saying that the single most frequent symptom of diabetes is the urge to have to go the bathroom to pee many times during the day since the body will try to evacuate some of the excess sugar through the urine[34]. Fatigue and blurred vision at certain times are other symptoms.

But don't get scared for nothing. Ask your medical doctor to do a full test and he/she will be able to tell you if you're blood sugar levels are normal or too high/too low. Remember that the human body is quite strong, it's only after many years of abuse that the pancreas cells just "burnout". So even if you are over 50 years old and have high sugar levels, proper nutrition and exercise (which will be explained further in this book), can help you reset your body to a certain extent and avoid diabetes as well as other conditions.

3.1.2. A few more words on simple carbs vs. complex carbs

There are some widespread measures when talking about carbs. So here are a few words on the notions on the glycemic index and on the glycemic load index.

---

[34] The urine of a person with non treated diabetes will taste sweet, in the sense "sugary". Lol another involuntary wordplay.

Glycemic index (GI)

The glycemic index (GI) is a measure of how quickly a carbohydrate is broken down into glucose. The GI goes from 0 to 100. Water which has no sugar will have a GI of 0, while refined sugar will have a GI of 100.

Glycemic load (GL)

The glycemic load (GL) is a measure of how much the blood sugar level will increase after one consumes a certain type of food. The GL basically takes the glycemic index of the carbohydrate found in the food and multiplies it by the quantity of carbohydrates in the food. Sounds complicated? Yeah, because it's hard to explain and I suck at writing. So let me give you an example and you will see how easy and intuitive the GL is.

Watermelon contains several types of sugar molecules (sucrose, glucose and fructose) which have a high glycemic index of approximately 72. However, since watermelon contains mostly water and only very little sugar, the glycemic load will be very low. In other words, the "quantity" of sugar in the watermelon is so low, that even if the types of sugar molecules contained in the watermelon go quickly in the blood stream, if one eats a watermelon, the blood sugar levels will only increase very moderately.

In numbers, this is the way we would calculate the glycemic load of the consumption of a 100gr watermelon (knowing that the glycemic index of the sugar in the watermelon is 72 and that 100gr of watermelon has approx 5gr of sugar).

GL = 5 x 72 /100 = 3.6

Below I posted a table on some of the GI and GL numbers of some foods.

Food Values: Glycemic Index/Glycemic Load

	Low GI	Med GI	High GI
Low GL	All-bran cereal (8,42) Apples (6,38) Carrots (3,47) Peanuts (1,14) Strawberries (1,40) Sweet Corn (9,54)	Beets (5,64) Cantaloupe (4,65) Pineapple (7,59) Sucrose, i.e. table sugar (7,68)	Popcorn (8,72) Watermelon (4,72) Whole wheat flour bread (9,71)
Med GL	Apple juice (11,40) Bananas (12,52) Fettucine (18,40) Orange juice (12,50) Sourdough wheat bread (15,54)	Life Cereal (16,66) New potatoes (12,57) Wild rice (18,57)	Cheerios (15,74) Shredded wheat (15,75)
High GL	Linguine (23,52) Macaroni (23,47) Spaghetti (20,42)	Couscous (23,65) White rice (23,64)	Baked Russet potatoes (26,85) Cornflakes (21,81)

Source: Revised International Table of Glycemic Index (GI) and Glycemic Load (GL), *The American Journal of Clinical Nutrition*, July 2002

Source: American Journal of Clinical Nutrition, July 2002

Of course, the higher the glycemic load index, the bigger the insulin response as the body gets in "panic mode" and has to eliminate as fast as possible, and in "any old way", the excess sugar from the blood.

Most GL indexes are in between (10 and 20) but it's *totally* wrong to base one's nutrition or diet on GI or GL indexes unless one has diabetes. Indeed we need a lot of energy to live, so forget about living on a diet eating just apples or raw carrots as you will not get enough calories from that. Moreover, when considering a healthy diet, other matters need to be considered including minerals and other nutrients, fibers, etc. For example rice, which has a high GL and mid GI index may seem as something to avoid. Wrong! Not only does it have a lot of energy, but the fibers found in rice and also help digestion, etc.

Therefore knowing the GI/GL of foods is interesting, but unless you are diabetic these measures are not useful for your nutrition. GI and

GL indexes are often publicized and sometimes even used in certain diets but as long as you exclude the real bad stuff on a regular basis[35] like sodas, pizzas, white bread, chips, etc, which have both very high GL and GI you will be doing okay. Indeed, if our food sources had low GL/GI indexes we would need to spend hours eating. Imagine how many watermelons a day we would need to eat if it were our only source of sugars. This also explains why the mammals that feed mainly on vegetable spend most of their days eating[36].

3.2. Other functions of carbs

Carbs are not only used as an immediate source of energy. Saccharide chains are also used in the frame of biological processes including the immune system and fertility for women. Here again you can see that some of the "nutrients" painted as "evil" by many dieting "experts" are simply *necessary* to stay alive and reproduce.

3.3. Lactose intolerance

Since there are quite a few people who are lactose intolerant, I want to say a few words on the subject. Carbs can be found in many foods/drinks. In the case of milk the carbs are called lactose. They are then broken down into glucose and galactose in the small intestine (in the duodenum[37]) by enzymes called lactase. Approximately 20% of the population is said to be lactose intolerant. From a clinical point of view, these persons suffer from a deficit of lactase in their intestine. The deficit of lactase can have as origin an injury to the small intestine, usually during infancy. The more common cause of lactase deficit is genetic.

---

[35] Nothing wrong with having a once in a while a "food orgy" with soda/alcohol, pizza, plenty of chips with yummy barbecue sauce and nachos with a thick guacamole sauce. But then again, just once in a while. And a "while" is measured in months, not days.

[36] They base their diet on very low glycemic food.

[37] The duodenum is the first part of the small intestine and comes right after the stomach.

Managing lactose intolerance is not difficult in modern society as one can find products especially made for those with a deficit of lactase. Interesting to note that the type of milk that has the highest percentage of lactose is human breast milk with around 9%. Yogurts can often be eaten by those with lactose intolerance, despite the high lactose content, as the bacteria used to make the yogurt will produce lactase which is then found in the yogurt and which helps the absorption of lactose. The lactose percentages in diary products commonly found are in the table below.

Dairy product	Serving size	Lactose content	Percentage
Milk, regular	250 ml	12 g	4.80%
Milk, reduced fat	250 ml	13 g	5.20%
Yogurt, plain, regular	200 g	9 g	4.50%
Yogurt, plain, low-fat	200 g	12 g	6.00%
Cheddar cheese	30 g	0.02 g	0.07%
Cottage cheese	30 g	0.1 g	0.33%
Butter	1 tsp (5.9ml)	0.03 g	0.51%
Ice cream	50 g	3 g	6.00%

Source: Wikipedia

Chapter 4: Vitamins, minerals and dietary fibers

Vitamins and minerals are among the best known nutrients and most people take multi-vitamin and mineral pills. However, the number of different vitamins and minerals is huge and their various uses in the human body are less well known.

4.1. Vitamins

Vitamins are classified as either water-soluble or fat-soluble. For humans there are 13 essential vitamins: 4 fat-soluble (A, D, E, and K) and 9 water-soluble (8 B vitamins and vitamin C). Because vitamins are not as easily stored as other nutrients, a consistent intake is important which is why a good nutrition is important. As said above, the fat-soluble vitamins are absorbed through the intestinal tract with the help of lipids.

Vitamins have diverse biochemical functions. Some regulate cells and tissues (e.g., some forms of vitamin A), others function as antioxidants[38] (e.g., vitamin E and vitamin C). The B vitamins are used, among others, to help enzymes catalyze certain reactions.

A lack of vitamins can lead to many diseases or disorders. This is why balanced diets are recommended. Multi-vitamin pills such as those sold in pharmacies can also help balance the body's needs. It is true that any excess of vitamin in the body can also create problems, but the dosages to reach to get in that problem area are quite high. So most people eating normally and taking the recommended dosage of their "multi-vitamin pill should be doing quite fine.

---

[38] As said above, anti-oxidants help prevent or limit the occurrence risk of many diseases including cancer, inflammatory bowel diseases, atherosclerosis, etc. So getting your daily suggested requirement of vitamins E and C are very important. Vitamins E and C can be found in many fruits and vegetables. This will be discussed later in the book.

4.1.1. Short description of some of the vitamins and their uses

Here is a short description of the vitamins and their uses in the human body. Since we see these vitamins in many of the food labels we eat, it's useful to understand some of their basics.

Vitamin A

Known as *retinol,* it's involved in healthy bone growth, as well as cell division. It helps regulate the immune system. It is also a key molecule for vision

Vitamin B1

Known as *thiamine,* it's essential in converting foods into energy, it supports the normal function of the nervous system, muscles and heart.

Vitamin B2

Known as *riboflavin,* it supports energy production. It's necessary for red blood cell and antibody production, respiration and regulating human growth and reproduction. It is essential for thyroid activity and tissue repair.

Vitamin B3

Known as *niacin,* it's primarily involved into converting food into energy. It regulates circulation, hormone production, the digestive and nervous systems, and promotes healthy skin. It's effective to increase levels of HDL (good) cholesterol.

Vitamin B5

Known as *pantothenic acid,* it helps the conversion of fat and sugar into energy.

Vitamin B6

Known as *pyridoxine,* it's necessary to balance the hormonal changes in women, assists in the growth of new cells and the functioning of the immune system. It's also involved in cancer immunity, red blood cell production, preventing skin problems and in fighting certain heart difficulties.

Vitamin B7

Known as *biotine,* it's involved in the metabolism (conversion) of fats and the production of fatty acids. It also helps keep a steady blood sugar level.

Vitamin B9

Known as *folic acid*, it's used in to create and repair DNA. It is also important in aiding rapid cell division both for adults and children. It is therefore a critical molecule during pregnancy.

Vitamin B12

Contains *cobalt* and is also known as *cobalamin.* The primary functions are to maintain a healthy nervous system and to produce red blood cells. Cobalamin is also involved in the synthesis (formation) of DNA.

Vitamin C

Known as a*bsorbic acid.* The human body is unable to store vitamin C which is why it needs to be taken on a regular basis. Vitamin C is important in forming collagen that gives structure to bones, cartilage, muscle and blood vessels. It also helps the absorption of iron and is a powerful antioxidant.

Vitamin D

The source of this vitamin is best known as being from sunlight, or more accurately, as being made in the body by exposure to UV rays. Vitamin D helps maintain adequate calcium and phosphor levels in the blood. It is also involved in regulating cell growth and maintaining a healthy immune system.

Vitamin E

These are a powerful source of antioxidants. They are also involved in the immune system, DNA repair, the protection of blood cells, the nervous system, muscles and the eye retina.

Vitamin K

This vitamin plays an essential role in the production of coagulation proteins, and the ability of blood to clot.

4.2. Minerals

Dietary minerals (also known as mineral nutrients) are the chemical elements required by living organisms, other than the "big four" elements (carbon, hydrogen, nitrogen, and oxygen) found in most organic molecules.

The minerals used in the human body include the seven "major" minerals which we have in abundance: calcium, phosphorus, potassium, sulfur, sodium, chlorine, and magnesium.

There are the "minor" minerals which are just as important for life but which we have in much smaller quantities. These include iron, cobalt, copper, zinc, molybdenum, iodine, and selenium.

Of course, these minerals have to be absorbed by the body as they cannot be created. In some cases bacteria will play an essential role in making the minerals "absorbable" by the body. For example, cobalt can only be used by the body once it has been transformed by bacteria into vitamin B12 which is used by all living cells in the frame of DNA processes and which plays a key role in the functioning of the brain.

Iron is the most known mineral as it is used by many proteins, including hemoglobin. Like all minerals in the body, too much or not enough of iron can cause health issues. Iron-deficiency anemia is a common anemia (low red blood cell level) caused by insufficient dietary intake and absorption of iron, and/or iron loss from bleeding. This is a frequent condition for women due to their periods. In most cases increasing the intake of food containing iron helps restore a good iron level in the body. It is interesting to note that vitamin C helps the absorption of iron by the body. So if you're a woman and are a little bit low on iron, taking dried meat (which contains a lot of iron) with orange juice (which has vitamin C) can prove quite effective if taken on a regular basis (1-2x/week). Here again, only a blood test done with your medical doctor will let you know how you stand with regards to iron[39].

It is well known that calcium is important for bones to avoid osteoporosis. But most people don't realize that calcium is also a key factor in the electrical conduction system of the heart as calcium will cause muscle contraction in the frame of the heart's electrical conduction system.

Potassium is also important in the heart electrical conduction system as it will prevent muscle contraction. It is the combination of calcium and potassium in the electric signals that will make sure that the heart contracts and then relaxes while getting filled with blood. Potassium is also very important in the neurological system and in keeping a good balance in the interstitial fluid which is the liquid in between cells.

Phosphor is, with calcium, the mineral that the body has in greatest quantity. Phosphates are a component of the DNA chains and phosphor is part of the ATP molecule. As reminder, ATP is the energy source at cellular level.

I will not go through all minerals, so I will end by saying that many are used in enzymes, including the antioxidant enzymes. Others,

---

[39] Only big iron deficiencies may require the intake of iron supplements through pills or injections.

such as iodine are used in the production on hormones (iodine being used for the thyroid hormones).

4.3. A few words on salt (NaCl)

Salt is an essential molecule for the good functioning of the human body. Too little salt or too much salt can put the body at risk. Among others, salt is necessary in many neurological processes. It enables a right balance of fluids in the body and enables the contraction and relaxation of muscles.

The kidneys naturally balance the amount of sodium stored in your body for optimal health. When your sodium levels are low, your kidneys essentially hold on to the sodium. When sodium levels are high, your kidneys excrete the excess in urine. But if for some reason your kidneys can't eliminate enough sodium, the sodium starts to accumulate in your blood. Because sodium attracts and holds water, your blood volume increases. Increased blood volume makes your heart work harder to move more blood through your blood vessels, which increases pressure in your arteries (i.e. high blood pressure).

This is why too much salt increases cardiovascular diseases. High salt intakes also can lead to stomach cancer and renal diseases. They can also provoke an enlargement of the left ventricle of the heart (condition known as cardiac enlargement) which can be a serious condition.

Salt contains approx 40% of sodium. The recommended salt levels are up to 5 grams per day, which equals to 2gr of sodium per day. A tablespoon of salt contains about 2.3grams of sodium so this shows you how little salt the body really needs. Since many processed and prepared foods have added salt, the average person in the developed countries will absorb well over 3gr of sodium per day (i.e. 50% more than the recommended quantity)!

In many Asian countries too, salt consumption is high. One tablespoon of traditional soy sauce has about 1gr of sodium.

This is why in the nutrition section of this book, I advise to avoid salt while cooking and to use other flavor enhancers such as lemon.

4.4. A few words on dietary fibers

Dietary fibers are totally unrelated to vitamins or minerals. I included them in this chapter as because I didn't know where else to put them and I don't feel like writing a whole chapter on them.

Dietary fibers are basically the indigestible portion of food derived from plants (vegetables, fruits). They can be water soluble or non water soluble.

4.4.1. Soluble fibers

Soluble fibers will dissolve in water and will ferment in the colon into gases and into byproducts which are useful for the body. They are prebiotic[40], which means that they stimulate the growth and activity of bacteria which are useful for the digestive system and beneficial to the overall health. Basically the fibers are the "food" for the bacteria in the human flora. This is why soluble fibers are vital although they are not absorbed by the human body. Do remember that in humans, bacteria play an essential role in the digestive system[41]. As a matter of fact, there are 10 times more bacteria in a human body than there are cells, mostly situated in the human flora.

Soluble fibers will attract water and form a viscous gel during the digestion which provides a sense of satiety which reduces further food intake. By doing so, fibers enable the body to absorb the

---

[40] Do not mistake prebiotic which are foods/substances that stimulate bacteria growth and activity with a probiotic which is a bacteria which is ingested to treat certain conditions. The ingestion of certain bacteria (probiotics) is used to treat/or has been shown to help in certain conditions including lactose intolerance, colon cancer, diarrhea, irritable bowel syndrome, blood pressure and cholesterol.

[41] Bacteria play also vital roles for plants as they are the organisms than are able to fix nitrogen from the atmosphere into the ground where the roots from plants will then absorb them. So remember, not all bacteria are evil. Without bacteria, there wouldn't be any vegetation. Without vegetation there wouldn't be any animal life.

nutrients taken. Without this sense of satiety, we would continue eating and our bodies wouldn't be able to absorb all the nutrients which would come in the blood flow. This would lead to very high (and fatal over time) levels of sugars and fatty acids.

Soluble fibers also have an impact on lowering total cholesterol and LDL cholesterol.

4.4.2. Non soluble fibers

By definition, non soluble fibers will not dissolve in water. However they also will ferment and have a prebiotic role. Non soluble fibers will tend to bulk by absorbing water as they more through the digestive system. As such they will accelerate the movement of food though the intestines by bulking the stool[42] and make it softer. Insufficient absorption of water and fibers is the most common source for constipation.

4.4.3. Other health benefits of fibers

Fibers do not bind to vitamins or metals and therefore do not limit their absorption. However they do facilitate the absorption of minerals, especially calcium. As said previously, in some cases the absorption of certain minerals is difficult and requires one or several "facilitators" to be absorbed by the body. Fibers play this role either directly or though the byproducts which are produced during their fermentation. Some of the main byproducts are short fatty acid chains which are involved in many vital mechanisms (non exhaustive list):

- They help regulate the acidity (pH) of the intestinal tract and therefore reduce the risk of colorectal cancer,

---

[42] The composition of feces is approx. 75% water and the remaining being unfermented fibers, bacteria from the human flora as well as other excreted elements.

- They help stabilize glucose levels by acting on the pancreas (insulin release) and the liver (glycogen breakdown),

- They help stimulate the production of cells and molecules involved in the immune system (T-helper cells, antibodies, leukocytes, cytokines, etc),

- They help improve the barrier properties of the colonic mucosal barrier which helps inhibit inflammatory and adhesion irritants (see chapter 5.5.). This is why a good fiber intake is advised for people diagnosed with irritable bowel syndrome, ulcerative colitis or Cohn's disease. These diseases are autoimmune diseases whereby the body's own immune system attacks elements of the digestive system.

The recommended fiber consumption of dietary fiber per day is 20-35 grams per day for an adult.

Lose weight now!

Part 2: Understanding the basics of the human body

Okay, now that you have understood the basics of the different nutrients (or that you have skipped part 1 which is a really *bad* idea), we need to get into the basics of the human body. Of course, this part can also be skipped too or read after if you want to get directly in the dieting chapters. However while this section may seem a bit geeky/medical and a little bit far from dieting, it's important for you to understand well how lifestyle and nutrition habits can affect positively or negatively some of the main functions of the body.

It's only by truly understanding the link between lifestyle choices, nutrition and health that one can understand why some things should be done and others not. This will also give you more motivation to go through the journey that will bring you to the physique and health condition you truly want.

But don't worry, this is not going to be an in-depth medical school course on anatomy. I am not going to focus on all the functions of the body, but only on the following two "systems" that are really directly affected by our lifestyle choices:

1. Cardio-pulmonary system (heart and lungs),
2. Musculoskeletal system (includes bones, muscles, tendons and ligaments).

Lose weight now!

Chapter 5: The heart

The cardio-pulmonary system is composed of the lungs and the heart. It's this system that takes the oxygen from the air you breathe and puts it in the blood stream. The heart functions as a pump ensuring that the flow of blood transporting oxygen and other nutrients to the cells is adapted to the body's needs.

5.1. Basic heart anatomy

Of all organs, the heart is the most important after the brain. The embryonic heart will actually start beating during the fourth weak after conception, and during the human life span it may beat over 3 billion times! The outer wall of the human heart is composed of three layers. The outer layer is called the epicardium. The middle layer is called the myocardium[43] and is composed of cardiac muscle which contracts. The inner layer is called the endocardium and is in contact with the blood that the heart pumps.

The human heart has four chambers, two superior atria and two inferior ventricles. The atria are the receiving chambers and the ventricles are the discharging chambers. The ventricles are those that actually "pump". The atrium and ventricles are separated by valves which ensure that the blood flow only goes in one direction. For the same purpose there is also one valve in between the right ventricle and the pulmonary artery, as well as another in between the left ventricle and the aorta.

The blood flow functions the following way. The deoxygenated blood (i.e. the one charged with carbon dioxide (CO_2), will get into the right atrium and then in the right ventricle which will pump this blood in the pulmonary artery, which will end in the numerous

---

[43] The myocardial infarction which is commonly known as "heart attack" will be discussed later.

capillaries in the lung where oxygen will get into the blood while the CO_2 goes back in the lungs where it will then be expired. Oxygen filled blood will then get into the left atrium and left ventricle before being pumped to the aorta and the rest of the body. The image below helps illustrate this.

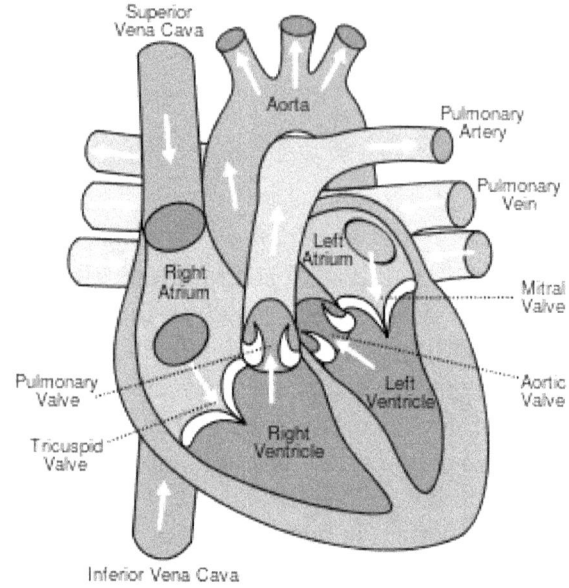

Source: Wikipedia

5. 2. The electrical conduction system of the heart

The heart beat is based on its own electrical system which is only dependant of the autonomic nervous system (ANS), also called involuntary nervous system. The ANS functions below the level of consciousness and controls the visceral functions. This is why the human body can continue working while we are sleeping or if we are unconscious.

The electric system in the heart works with a system of nerves and its purpose is that all the muscle cells of the heart beat in a coordinated way at the same time, while respecting a certain pattern. There are 3 main parts to the electric system.

1) Sinoatrial node (SA node): the SA node is located in the upper part of the right atrium. This is where the cardiac neurons start emitting the electric signal.

2) Atrioventrical node (AV node): the AV node is located just beside the valve separating the right atrium and the right ventricle

3) Purkinje Fibers and the bundle branches. These are the nerve ramifications which go from the AV node to the heart's myocardium

The images below help illustrate this.

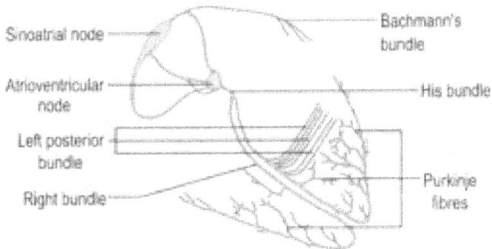

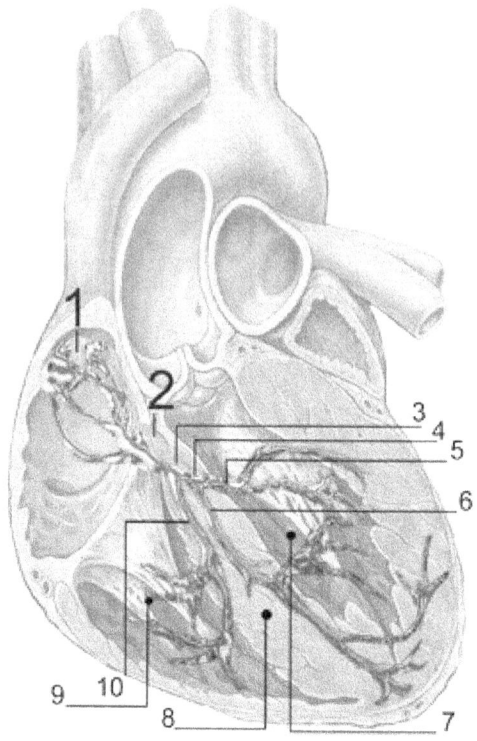

1. Sinoatrial node	6. Left posterior fascicle
2. Atrioventrical node	7. Left ventricle
3. Bundle of His	8. Ventricular septum
4. Left bundle branch	9. Right ventricle
5. Left anterior fascicle	10. Right bundle branch

Source: Wikipedia

The electric signal works as follows. The SA node generates a signal that will lead both atria to contract and push the blood in the ventricles. The AV node will delay the SA node's signal to the rest of the nerves. This delay is necessary to avoid that both the atria and ventricles contract at the same time. Once the electrical signal has been delayed by the AV node it will then go the Purkinke Fibers and bundle branches, causing the ventricles (through stimulation of all myocardial muscle cells) to contract. For information, the total time taken by the nerve impulse in the heart to go from its starting point to its end point is 0.19 seconds. Once this cycle has ended, the ventricles are repolarized and the cycle repeats. The complex mechanisms of the electric signals involving calcium and potassium ions will not be explained in this book. Therefore, if you are a total nerd and have no life at all, please have an enjoyable week-end by yourself reading about how this works. You will find everything you need on internet. Even the name of a psychologist to help treat you.

5.3. Electrical conduction disorders (cardiac dysrhythmia)

For a resting heart, the impulse that originates from the SA node is at a relative frequency of 60-100 beats per minute (bpm). This is known as the normal sinus rhythm. If the SA nodal impulses are below 60bpm the there is a condition known as bradycardia. If the SA nodal impulses are above 100bpm, there is a condition known as tachycardia.

5.3.1. Bradycardia

Bradycardia may cause not enough oxygen to be pumped into the heart. It can lead to fainting, shortness of breath, or even death if really severe. Bradycardia can be caused, among others, by disorders in the SA node or the AV node, diseases of the cardiac valves, hormonal issues or the use/abuse of recreational drugs. Some medicines treating high blood pressure can also cause lead to bradycardia (e.g. beta-blockers).

The best way to identify bradycardia is through an electrocardiogram (ECG) by a doctor. Of course, measuring your pulse when at rest is the easiest and first way to start the diagnosis process. So clearly if your pulse is below 60, ask your doctor for an ECG. The other symptoms of bradycardia include feeling tired, having short breath, being dizzy or having chest pains. Since these symptoms tend to go fairly unnoticed having an ECG is really the best thing.

Bradycardia is usually treated though a change in diet, changes in medication or specific medical drugs. In some cases it is necessary to get a pacemaker which will provide to the heart the electrical stimulus that it lacks.

5.3.2. Tachycardia

Tachycardia can be caused by various factors. However, tachycardia can be dangerous depending on the speed and type of rhythm that the heart follows. It's interesting to note that while tachycardia for adults starts with heart beats of over 100bpm, the number is quite different for children whose normal heart beats are much lower than those adults. For example babies have normal heart beats up to 160bpm while 5 year old children will have normal heart beats of up to 130bpm. 12 year olds will have normal heart beats of up to 120bpm. So do keep this in mind if you are taking the pulse of a kid and don't worry right away about the kid having tachycardia.

As for bradycardia, the best way to identify tachycardia is through an electrocardiogram (ECG) by a doctor. As above, measuring your pulse when at rest is the easiest and first way to start the diagnosis process. The symptoms of tachycardia are similar to those of bradycardia and include having short breath, being dizzy, heart palpitations (racing or irregular heartbeat, uncomfortable sensation), chest pain, fainting. Again, only an ECG can provide a definite diagnosis.

There are many causes for tachycardia and an ECG is the best way to identify the cause(s). There are two big groups of tachycardia: sinus tachycardia and ventricular tachycardia.

Sinus tachycardia is when there is an increase in the autonomic nervous system (ANS) stimulation to the heart. As said above, the ANS is the part of the nervous system that manages the vital organs without that we need to "think about it". For example, a chemical or hormonal disorder may lead the body to produce more adrenaline than what is really needed.

However *external substances* to the body may also lead to sinus tachycardia. Stimulants such as caffeine, nicotine, as well as drugs such as amphetamines or cocaine will also enhance the activity of the ANS and can cause or aggravate sinus tachycardia as they will also tend to increase the heartbeat. They can also provoke irregular rhythm. The consumption of caffeine and stimulants at high dosages, such as found in energy drunks, has been linked to deaths. Avoiding abuses of alcohol is also recommended as alcohol can also aggravate certain forms of tachycardia.

In the case that sinus tachycardia is due to imbalances *within the body*, some medications can help treat the problem. Medications can include anti-arrhythmic drugs or drugs to block some of the thyroid hormones.[44] An increase of potassium consumption[45] can also sometimes be recommended since potassium is involved in the phase when the heart does not contract. Of course avoiding stimulants such as coffee, soda drinks or recreational drugs is necessary.

For sinus tachycardia related to the consumption of *external substances*, or a condition where the body is very sensitive to external stimulants, avoiding stimulants such as coffee, soda drinks or recreational drugs is necessary. Sometimes increasing the consumption of potassium can also be helpful.

Potassium levels can be checked in the frame of blood tests.

Ventricular tachycardia (V-tach) is a condition where the arrhythmia (irregular electric signal) originates in the ventricles. Rather than having a normal electric signal going from the SA node to the AV node and then to the Purkinje Fibers and the bundle branches, there will be additional electric signals which will be generated directly in the ventricle. These "parasite" signals will conflict with the "good" electrical signal and thus lead to more contractions than necessary and situations where the ventricle will contract even if it not totally filled with blood. V-tach is a life threatening condition.

---

[44] The thyroid hormones regulate the metabolism's speed. If these hormones are produced in to big quantities (hyperthyroidism), the body's metabolism will be too fast. This can include faster heart beats.
[45] Potassium rich foods will be discussed later in the diet section.

V-tach can be treated in certain cases by medications, including anti-arrhythmic drugs such as beta blockers or calcium channel blockers. Another alternative is the catheter ablation which is an effective (not too intrusive) procedure. In this procedure a small catheter inserted through the blood vessel in the hip will go to the heart where it will neutralize through heat, cold, or radiofrequency energy the area of the ventricular which is at the origin of sending the parasite signals. This procedure is effective as it permanently destroys the tissue at the origin of the parasite signals. People who undergo this procedure are often able to return home the same day or one day after.

5.4. Heart diseases: myocardial infraction and cerebral vascular accident

The two most common causes for death are related to the heart. They are the myocardial infraction (MI) and the cerebral vascular accident (CVA). Diseases related to the heart's valves can also be deadly but will not be discussed in this book. As said in chapter 0, doing an ECG is the best way to make sure that you are healthy or that any heart issue be detected as quickly as possible to ensure its proper treatment.

The good news is that in the great majority of cases, heart issues which are detected before an "accident" can be treated effectively and will enable those who suffer from them to lead basically a very normal life. For those over 50 years old, regular blood tests, ECGs and discussions with your doctor are a highly recommended practice.

5.4.1. Myocardial infraction (MI)

The body's blood system is fairly well done. Blood will go to the body from point A to point B through several "parallel" blood vessels which are alternative routes to get from point A to point B. Therefore if one blood vessel is cut or blocked, the blood will be able to use another vessel to get to destination. This system with "alternative routes" unfortunately has an exception which is the heart. Heart myocardial cells are *only* feeded through the coronary arteries. Therefore, if the coronary arteries are blocked through atherosclerotic plague, the myocardial cells will not get sufficient oxygen which will cause them to die (there is no other blood vessel to supply them with the oxygen and nutrients they need). The myocardial cells which will die are those in the area where there is the oxygen shortage. If the area of dead myocardial cells is too big, the heart will basically not have enough muscle cells to "pump" anymore therefore triggering a myocardial infraction. In common language a myocardial infraction is known as a "heart attack". Bypass surgery and/or the use of stents to widen the blocked coronary arteries are the only remedies at that point.

The image below shows the right coronary artery (RCA) and the left coronary artery (LCA). The occlusion (marked by point 1), leads to the insufficient supply of oxygen to the myocardial cells of the region of the bottom of the heart. This area is marked by point 2.

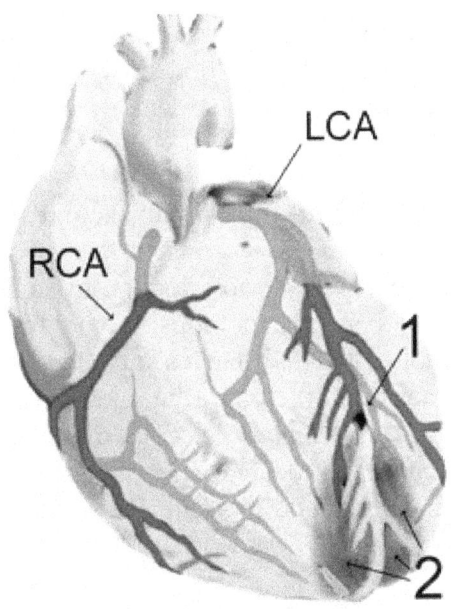

Source: Wikipedia

5.4.2. Cerebral vascular accident (CVA)

CVAs are similar to the myocardial infraction in the way they work. However rather than the coronary artery being blocked and depriving myocardial muscle cells from the oxygen they need, CVAs are when brain vessels are blocked and thus deprive neurons of a certain region of the brain of oxygen. Depending on the region of the "blockage", the consequences for the victim will be very different. CVA's are of course deadly as neurons will start to die after 3 minutes without oxygen and beyond 10 minutes without oxygen the survival rate is basically 0% in normal circumstances (i.e. not in hypothermia). In the case of CVAs, the blockage can be due to atherosclerosis (like for the myocardial infraction) or a clot which is basically some kind of "solid particle" which will block the blood stream.

Clots can have different origins and causes. There can be blood clots which are due to hemorrhages in some blood vessels. There can also be "fat" clots which can occur if part of an atherosclerotic plaque is removed by the pressure of the blood flow[46] from the blood vessel wall and re-injected into the blood stream.

5.4.3. Effects of smoking on the cardiovascular system

Okay, this is not a book about how to stop to smoke or why not to smoke. However it's simply obvious to me that you cannot be healthy if you smoke. The substances included in cigarettes are so dangerous that they can increase the likelihood of all kinds of diseases in a significant manner (e.g. >10x more chances of a getting a heart attack). Smoking decreases the capacity of the lung to exchange gas with the blood vessels, but let's focus here on the heart.

---

[46] This is one of the reasons why high blood pressure increases the risk of heart problems. Basically high blood pressure will tend to create blood vessel wall "erosion". This can lead to hemorrhages and blood clots going in the blood stream. It can also lead to "fat" clots formerly in the artery walls (endothelium) being re-injected in the blood stream.

As far as the cardiovascular system, smoking does provoke vasoconstriction (i.e. narrowing) of the blood vessels, thus leading to higher blood pressure whose consequences have been discussed above. In addition, narrower blood vessels have more chances of getting blocked by blood clots or fat clots. This is why smokers have such greater probabilities of getting fatal heart attacks or cerebral vascular accidents. As discussed below in section 5.5, smoke contains substances that will lead to an increase inflammatory response from the body. This state of inflammation is the source, as well as an aggravating factor, for several life threatening medical conditions.

If you're a guy under 90 years old, there is probably a more convincing reason for you to stop smoking. In two words: "limp dick"[47]. This is obvious as an inadequate blood circulation will eventually lead to the "spagettification[48]" of even Rocco Siffredi's[49] manhood.

So if you want to avoid a really embarrassing moment in bed with your girlfriend/boyfriend or whatever you have next to you[50], or if you don't want to end up a regular user of drugs against erectile dysfunction, stop smoking.

If you are a woman, of course you do not have this problem, but there are other risks besides the "usual" cancers, fetal malformations, pregnancy risks, etc, which are related to smoking.

It has been found that smoking increases the risk of painful or irregular periods, it advances menopause by an average of 2 years and reduces fertility. In addition, the vasoconstriction of the blood vessels around the vagina and clitoris can reduce the pleasure from sexual intercourse, thus leading to decreased feminine libido over

---

[47] Also known as the most embarrassing moment in a man's life. That's the moment when he thinks stuff like "shoot me now" or "I wish I had been born as a girl" while looking at the incredulous stare from his partner's eyes.
[48] For those that don't get it, it's the transformation of something as "hard as steel" into something as hard as an overcooked spaghetti.
[49] Somebody told me he is a famous Italian porn star. I don't know. I have never watched that sort of stuff...haha.
[50] As long as it's over 18 years old and consenting.

time. So here again, don't expect lasting fireworks in bed if you are a regular smoker.

Of course, people can do whatever they want. But if you smoke on a regular basis, there is no chance whatever that you'll ever be in good health, or as they say, it will freeze in hell before that happens. And to this date, there is no indication that the devil has asked for a radiator or a winter jacket.

5.5. An in-depth look at atherosclerosis for non medical professionals

In chapter 2, sections 2.1.1 and 2.2.2, I briefly went through the basics of atherosclerosis. I did mention the link in between fats and clogged arteries, but unfortunately things are much more complex in reality. Atherosclerosis is much more than just "fat" being "stored" in the walls of arteries. I know you are probably not a medical professional, but nevertheless the atherosclerosis process can be explained in easy words, especially that you now have some of the basics. Of course, you can skip this section if you don't want to get into more detail on atherosclerosis. You can also skip the whole book if you want. And as goes the saying: "if you don't like education, try ignorance". Still here? Great, now back to the nerdy stuff. ☺

5.5.1. Atherosclerosis for dummies

So here is a more detailed explanation on how the whole atherosclerosis process works.

Step 1: Oxidative stress related to food absorption

When food is ingested, the different macro-nutrients (lipids, carbs, and proteins) eventually go though the small intestine into the blood flow. As the blood flow "receives" a stream of "new molecules", the immune system, made of the white cells and other signal molecules, can get "activated". In the case that the quantity and/or combination of the macro-nutrients is not "balanced", this can lead to a state of "oxidative stress". Oxidative stress is a state where there is an "imbalance" in the oxygen contained in the molecules whereby there is a presence of "reactive oxygen species", i.e. free radicals.

The ingestion of saturated fatty acids, trans-fats, high levels of simple sugars will lead to a high state of oxidative stress. On the other hand, unsaturated fatty acids, or foods with a higher level of antioxidants will lead to a much lower oxidative stress situation. This is why, for example, one glass of red wine (with the anti-oxidants inside) can balance in the body simultaneous intake of a red meat filled with saturated fatty acids. This explains the relative "good" health of many French who tend to eat a lot of red meat. It's the intake of the anti-oxidants within the red wine that help offset the intake of the unhealthy saturated fatty acids[51].

Other non-food related factors which can increase oxidative stress include hereditary factors, as well as external factors (air pollution, stress) and lifestyle choices (other than food, this would include mainly level of physical activity, smoking and stress related to our daily lives[52]). While oxidative stress is well known for being a big

---

[51] A list of anti-oxidant foods and drinks will be provided later in the book.

[52] In some cases stress is due to external factors, in others it can come from lifestyle choices. Frequent professional traveling can be a source of lifestyle stress. From a workplace point of view, night shifts and irregular work hours are known to be causes of oxidative stress. Time pressures, if not properly managed, can also lead to stress. This is

factor for cancer and cardiovascular diseases, it's also a critical factor in other diseases such as Parkinson, Alzheimer. Oxidative stress is also thought to be a cause in many other neurological diseases[53].

Step 2: Immune reaction and inflammatory response

The oxidative stress situation will lead to an immune system response and therefore an inflammatory response[54]. Inflammation is the process whereby tissues swell in order, among others, to enable a faster flow of the white cells (leukocytes) as well as plasma towards the "site" where there is the inflammation. The inflammation process also facilitates the passage of molecules from one area to another (often from the blood to the cells). Inflammation is also the first step of healing.

In the case of the absorption of a meal with lots of simple sugars, saturated fatty acids, transfats and not enough foods with antioxidants, the white cells will start producing a chain of signaling molecules called "cytokins". Cytokins include the family of the "well-known" "interleukin" molecules.

A pro-oxidative meal ingested will therefore trigger a chain of reactions whereby many signaling molecules will be released in the blood stream with unintended consequences (see steps 3 and 4).

As said previously, smoking is not only dangerous for the lungs, but it also increases the state of inflammation in the body, therefore increasing oxidative stress in the body. A combination of an "unhealthy meal" with smoking basically doubles down the body's

---

why if you think that you can't handle the stress level associated to a certain activity, you shouldn't be doing it (if possible). In the cases where the professional stress factor is unavoidable (due to the nature of the job), then a focus on proper eating and exercising are vital as well as stress management techniques.

[53] This is why smoking, and its effect on the body's overall oxidative stress, can lead to many more medical conditions than "just" lung cancer or cardiovascular diseases.

[54] As said in chapter 4.4.3, dietary fibers help reduce the inflammatory response of the digestive system when there is an intake of food.

inflammatory state and therefore the consequences mentioned in steps 3 and 4 below.

Step 3: Endothelium dysfunction and atheroma

The endothelium is the inner wall of the blood vessels. Endothelium dysfunction is defined as the state whereby there is an imbalance in between vasodilatation (widening of the vessel) and vasoconstriction (narrowing of the vessel) due to substances produced or acting on the endothelium.

The release of signaling molecules due to a pro-oxidative meal will affect the endothelium of blood vessels and cause endothelium dysfunction. This will happen as they will increase "cell adhesion". As the name says, this will increase the probability that molecules (including the well-known LDL cholesterol, as well as other saturated fatty acids and transfats) get stuck to the cell of the endothelium, thus triggering an additional immune system response whereby white cells will be send to "eat" this "bad stuff". However, this has as consequence that 1) white cells start getting in the interior of the blood vessel and 2) once a "white cell" has "eaten" the molecular "bad stuff", the white cell will decompose and other white cells will be sent to "clean up" the mess. From a more chemical point of view, it's the oxidation of the LDL and other molecules which will cause the white cells to target them.

"Atheroma" is the name for the accumulation in artery walls of plague which is made up of (mostly) dead macrophage cells (white cells), other debris, lipids (cholesterol and fatty acids), calcium and a variable amount of "scar tissues" which make the artery wall even more fragile as scar tissue is not as "productive" as the "normal pre-wounded tissue". Scar tissue is also more fragile and is easier to tear and break-up.

As said before, when the atheroma becomes too big, there is a risk of "breaking up". If this happens, this releases in the blood stream the deposits of fat, etc. This is what is known as a "thrombosis". If large enough, the thrombosis [55] can block an artery and thus lead to a heart attack (blocked coronary artery), a cerebral vascular accident (blocked brain artery) or a pulmonary embolism (blocked lung artery). The risk of "breaking up" of the atheroma is related to its size and the blood pressure, since higher blood pressure will tend to damage the epithelium.

On the internet, you can find images of arteries with atheroma. It looks quite gross so I didn't put any image here in the book in order not to cut your appetite. But here's an image which illustrates the idea.

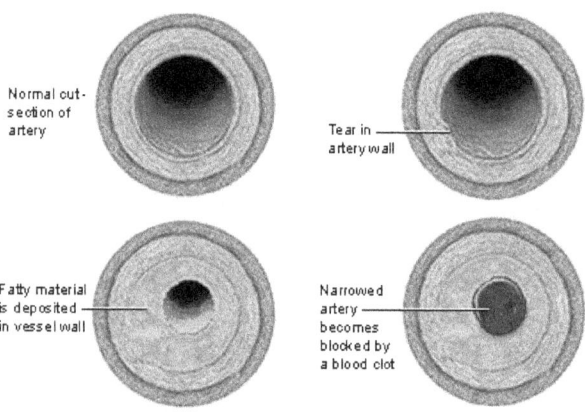

Source: unknown, internet

Step 4: Insulin resistance

The production of cytokins, other signaling molecules and enzymes tends to decrease the insulin response. In other words, the body is less effective at removing fast the excess sugars from the blood. Over time this increases the risk of diabetes as the pancreas cells are so solicited by producing insulin that one day they just stop working. The increase presence of excess sugars will then re-trigger an immune system and it's a vicious circle that begins.

Step 5: Liver LDL/HDL production

---

[55] Thromboses are generally treated through the injection of powerful anticoagulants.

The liver is a key organ in the body and basically filters and cleans the blood stream from toxins (alcohol, etc), non desirable elements (mercury) and excessive/non desirable molecules (saturated fatty acids). If the blood stream gets too many saturated fatty acids/transfats, the liver removes them from the body and re-uses them in the form of LDL cholesterol. As seen in step 3, LDL are molecules which will tend to adhere to the endothelium (artery wall) in the area where there is the inflammation (which is basically the whole arterial system as the blood stream is everywhere).

5.5.2. Why is there no atherosclerosis in veins?

Cool, I finished writing the section on atherosclerosis and stuff. I can soon go to bed. However before that I would like to explain shortly why atherosclerosis cannot happen in veins. Indeed as you may have noticed, we have only focused on arteries thus far.

There are basically two reasons why atherosclerosis cannot occur in veins. Firstly, the veins tend to be much thinner with less muscle around them than arteries. This is because the blood pressure they face is lower. Since they have less muscles to "vasodilate" or "vasoconstrict" to manage the blood flow, veins are endowed with valves which enable blood to go in only one way (see image below). Since veins are thinner, with less muscle fiber, there is of course less space for fat/debris building up within the endothelium of veins.

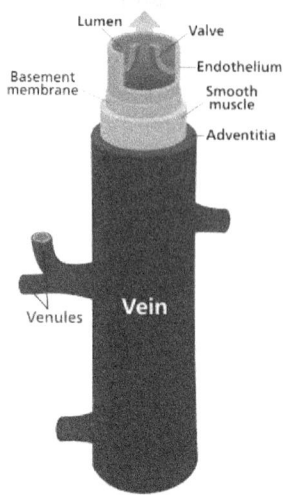

Source: Wikipedia

Second, and this is by far the most important reason, since veins have little oxygen in them (by definition, as the oxygen was given to the cells and the veins mainly transport CO2), there can be no oxidation. Therefore LDLs, saturated fatty acids, transfats and company are not oxidized in veins. Consequently, there is no immune system reaction /inflammatory response in veins which therefore do not suffer from atherosclerosis.

However, a thrombosis/blood clot that originates from an artery can go in the blood flow into veins and block them, a condition which can also be fatal. So although the veins are not the source of the debris/fat deposits which constitutes the thrombosis, they can be blocked by them.

Deep vein thrombosis, renal vein thrombosis, jugular vein thrombosis are among the serious, life threatening conditions which can result from a thrombosis getting blocked in a specific vein.

5.5.3. The fallacy of the "each calorie is the same" speech

Last night I was listening to an interview given by the president of US operations for a big American soda company. He was asked about the obesity problem in the US. More specifically he was asked on whether he thought that the sugary drinks of his company were part of the problem.

Of course, like other "death dealers", he did not answer the question. He simply said that his company was encouraging people to do physical activities. He also argued that "one calorie is one calorie" and that as long as people do physical activities to burn the calories they will be doing okay.

Nothing is further from the truth than this statement. This is a lie.

Actually, he should be sued for issuing such statements. If the soda industry went the way of the tobacco industry, i.e. if it were defendant in class actions for concealing the health risks posed by regular consumption of their products, this executive's interview could serve as a piece of evidence to illustrate deceitful marketing practices. Here's why.

While a calorie is a calorie from an pure energy point of view, the body does not react in the same way if it receives 10 units of calories in one unit of time or if it gets these 10 units of calories over a period of 10 units of time.

Indeed, if the body receives these calories very quickly (which is the case for sweet sodas which have high levels of simple sugars), the biological reactions will be much greater than if the same number of sugars were received over a longer period of time. The higher insulin production, as well as the higher inflammatory state, will lead to faster and greater plague formation.

This is why 150kcal coming from an oatmeal breakfast are healthy for the body, while 150kcal coming from a sweet soda (or food with high saturated fatty acids) are unhealthy.

5.6. Heart muscle and physical activities

Physical activities such as sport will force the heart to pump more blood faster into the body. If physical activities are regular, this will lead to increasing the strength of the myocardial cells, thus making them gain volume (and thus the volume of the heart). Stronger hearts are able to pump more blood with a single beat, thus lowering the heart beats per minute. This is enviable as it will contribute to lower blood pressure. As said above, the higher the blood pressure, the greater the "erosion" of the walls of the blood vessels.

More on the benefits of physical activities and how they relate to the heart will be discussed later.

5.7. Cardiopulmonary resuscitation (CPR)

CPR is beyond the scope of this book. However since heart attacks/cerebral vascular accidents are frequent causes of death, everyone over 12 years old should be able to know how to perform CPR.

I'm not going to go into first aid stuff, but the basic steps are the following if you see an unconscious person who no longer breathes and whose heart has stopped (breathing stops after a few seconds when the heart no longer beats):

1) Call for help (paramedics or police).

2) Make sure you're in an area where there is no danger for your health (no fire, electricity or other risks) and where you can perform CPR safely.

3) Do compressions on the thorax at a rhythm of 100-120 compressions per minute. The compressions should be approx 4 cm deep on an adult so don't be afraid to do it strong. The compressions should be done at the intersection of the middle of the sternum (vertical line) and the middle of the pectoral muscles

(horizontal line). Compressions continue as long as you can perform them, if possible until medical help arrives.

Here is a really short (1'20) video I found on internet on how to perform CPR (basics):

http://www.youtube.com/watch?v=EGMSH7uz8kM
(Liverpool John Moores University)

Of course, if you want to learn more on CPR, or how to perform it on babies or children, check out the first aid courses available in your neighborhood.

Chapter 6: The lungs

Everybody knows about the lungs. Lungs are the sponge like organ which enables the exchange of oxygen in the blood and the carbon dioxide (CO_2) out of the blood. It is interesting to note that the lungs are to a certain extent "overbuilt" as their capacity is much greater than actually needed. One can actually live normally with only one lung. This is why smokers can smoke for years without noticing an impact on their lung functions.

6.1. Basic lung anatomy

The lung is like a sponge whereby there is a lot of "empty" space. The air that we inhale goes in the bronchi, which become smaller and smaller airways. At the smallest scale, the bronchioles are the airways that will get into contact with the alveoli whose grape-like shape are made of specialized cells where the exchange of oxygen and CO_2 takes place. The reason why smoking is bad for the lungs (and I'm not even going to get into the cancer part) is that the tar will end in the alveoli and therefore block the exchanges of gas in between the cells of the alveoli and the blood vessels.

The images below help illustrate this.

Bronchi, Bronchial Tree, and Lungs

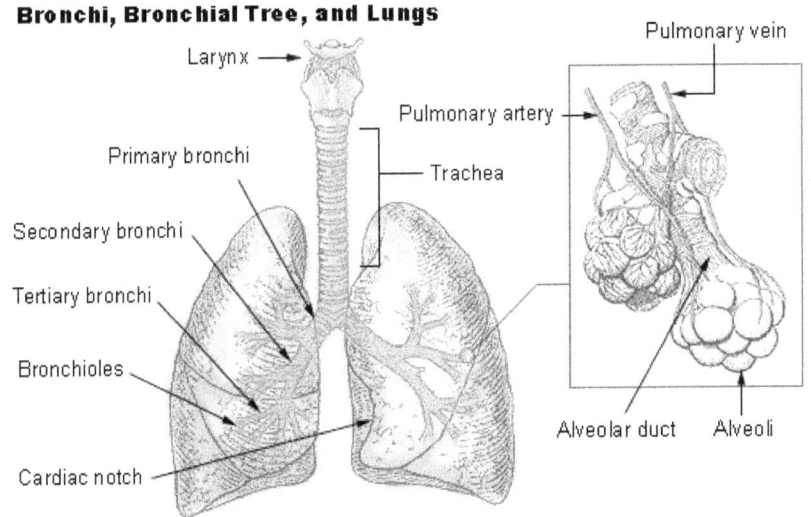

Source: Wikipedia

6.2. The thoracic diaphragm and the respiratory mechanism

The thoracic diaphragm (hereafter diaphragm) is the internal muscle that is necessary for the lungs to get filled with air, and then to empty the air. The diaphragm is just below the lungs. As this muscle contracts, it increases the volume of the thoracic cage, thus forcing air in the lungs. This is the inhalation part. On the other side, when the diaphragm relaxes, the volume in the thoracic cage decreases, thus forcing air out of the lungs. This is the expiration part.

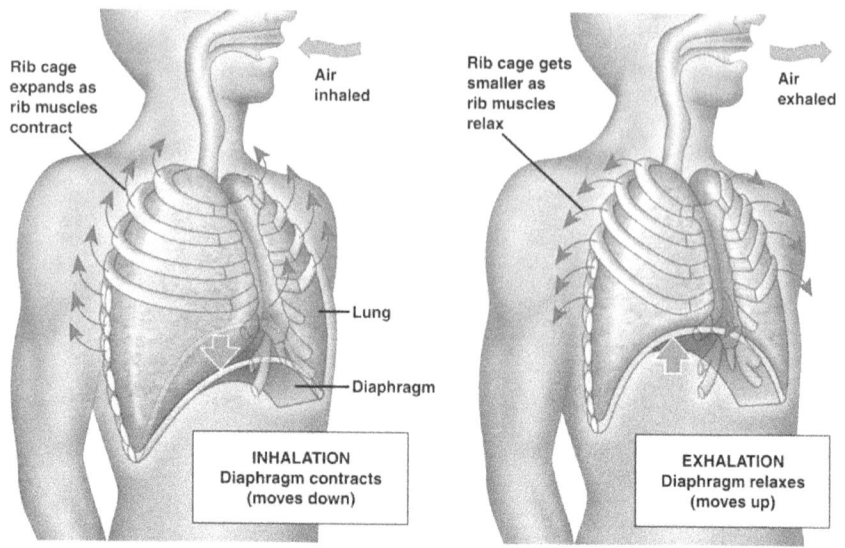

Source: unidentified web site found through Google images

6.3. Lung diseases: cancer and effects of smoking

I will only focus here on the cardio-vascular. I will not cover asthma which is another frequent condition related to the lungs (although more related to the immune system). For those interested on that topic, check out the internet.

Smoking decreases the capacity of the lung to exchange gas with the blood vessels at the level of the alveoli which is why smokers eventually are totally out-of-breath, but let's focus on cancer.

In short, certain substances of tobacco smoke can provoke uncontrolled tissue growth in the lung. Even passive smoking still poses the threat of lung cancer which is why passive smoking and restricting smoking to certain public areas is slowly being implemented in developed countries.

I won't go more into detail into lung cancer. I will just say that the survival rate after 5 years after being diagnosed with lung cancer is less than 15%. Amen.

6.4. The lung, the diaphragm muscle and physical activities

Physical activities such as sport will also increase the strength of the diaphragm. A stronger diaphragm will be able to contract more thus enabling to inhale a greater quantity of air in a single breath.

Physical activities also increase lung volumes and increase the effectiveness of gas exchange at cellular level (alveoli). This will be discussed later in greater detail.

Chapter 7: The bones

As the body is mostly made of water, it is the musculoskeletal system that enables humans to stand on our feet and that gives us shape. The musculoskeletal system includes bones, muscles, tendons and ligaments. All shall be discussed here. I will also talk about joints/articulations and back problems as they are common sources of pain despite the fact that they can be to a certain extent avoided.

7.1. Bones

7.1.1. Bone functions

Bones are the rigid organs that make the skeleton of humans. They support and protect the various organs of the body. For example the ribs will protect the thoracic cage while the skull will protect the brain. The bones also enable us to move. It is interesting to know that babies are born with over 270 bones, but with time some of them fuse together which leads adults to have 206 separate bones.

It is within the marrow of the long bones that red and white cells are produced. Bones also serve as storage areas. They can store minerals such as calcium and phosphor, but also fatty acids, heavy metals as well as foreign elements which can be harmful to other tissues. Bones also have other functions, including the one of helping to keep the blood pH[56] relatively stable.

Bone tissue is always being replaced in a process called bone remodeling. Throughout one's life, mature bone tissue is removed (bone resorption) while new bone tissue is formed (ossification). In the first year, a baby will replace almost 100% of his skeleton.

---

[56] The pH measures the acidity or basicness of a liquid.

In adults, the remodeling process still represents about 10% of all bones!

An imbalance in between the bone resorption process and the bone formation process is at the origin of many bone diseases, including osteoporosis.

7.1.2. Bone diseases: a look at osteoporosis

Osteoporosis is the most frequent bone disease and is worth while discussing in a book related to overall health.

Osteoporosis is a bone disease that leads to an increased risk of fractures due to the reduction of the bone mineral density. There are two types of this disease: primary type 1 and primary type 2.

Primary type 1 is the form of osteoporosis related to women after menopause. Primary type 2 is the form of osteoporosis seen in both males and females after age 75. However even in type 2, women are more affected than men by a factor of 2:1.

Both types 1 and type 2 are affected by a decrease in hormone production (estrogens for females, and testosterone for males). This decrease will negatively affect the bone formation process, which will therefore be insufficient to compensate the bone resorption process.

There are no symptoms for osteoporosis. Therefore women and older persons should consult with their doctor to do periodical radiographies which is the best way to identify this disease.

7.1.3. Preventing osteoporosis and other bone diseases

While there are hereditary predispositions, there are ways to try to prevent osteoporosis or to at least limit the speed at which the bone density loss will occur. Nutrition and lifestyle are the best prevention methods, together with specific medication in certain cases.

Physical activities will help delay bone degeneration as the "pressure" on bones will favor the bone formation processes. This is why overweight people are less at risk that skinny people when it comes to osteoporosis. The weight they have will have as mechanical consequence to stimulate the bone formation process to increase the bone density.

Furthermore, there is a strong relationship in between muscle mass and bone density. Thus stronger (and heavier) muscles will help keep bones strong.

As far as nutrition, both calcium and vitamin D are recommended for preventing/managing osteoporosis.

To the opposite, excess alcohol increases fracture risk. Tobacco smoking also is associated to decreased bone formation by affecting the cells involved in bone creation (called osteoblasts).

Physical exercises (good for the bones and other parts/functions of the body) will be discussed further in this book.

Chapter 8: Cartilage

Cartilage is a tissue which is found in many areas of the body, among others at the joints between bones. Cartilages do include collagen fibers to give them elasticity. It is important to know that cartilages do not have blood vessels and are supplied in nutrients by the blood vessels nearby.

At bone joints, the purpose of cartilage is to absorb shocks so not to have the bones touch other. This is why when you jump the bones are not going to hit each other (otherwise it would hurt a lot). As such they serve as a protective cushion.

Cartilage also enables a fluid mobility of the bones at the articulation. They are thus very important tissues for human mobility and therefore quality of life.

8.1. Cartilage diseases

Unfortunately, cartilage has limited repair capabilities as the cells which form it are not mobile and because it does not have a blood supply of its own.

So unlike other body parts, once cartilage gets too badly damaged or worn, it does not heal properly and there is a very high risk of developing osteoarthritis over time. This then becomes a chronic and permanent condition which explains why prevention is so important.

8.1.1. Osteoarthritis (or degenerative arthritis)

The most common cartilage diseases is osteoarthritis (also called as degenerative arthritis)

Osteoarthritis is basically the ossification of the cartilage tissue. This can be due to the cartilage being worn out over time or ruptures/ detachment (often due to sport injury).

Since the cartilage cannot fix itself, surgery if often the only alternative for important articulations such as knee, shoulder or back.

8.1.2. Spinal disc hernia and spinal disc degeneration

In the back, the spinal discs are the "cushion" which is located in between each vertebra. They are made of fibers of cartilage-like tissue. In the case of too much weight (e.g. when lifting a weight which is too heavy) or the case of an injury (car accident), the pressure on the spinal disc may be so big that the disc will flatten or get deformed.

If the person is young and the pressure not too big, the disc will recover its shape after a few days. However with age, and the repetition of shocks, the disc will recover less and less its shape. It will therefore tend to flatten.

For people with weaker discs, when there is too much pressure on the disc, the disc may not only flatten, in some cases it may rupture (disc hernia). When this occurs, the herniated disc (whose shape is no longer as "tight" as what it was) may start touching nerves. This is the cause for sciatics, and many other issues. As said before, since the cartilage cannot heal itself, surgery is the only option for herniated discs that start squeezing/touching nerves.

Spinal disc degeneration is the condition whereby the spinal disc just wears out. If the degeneration is too significant, the vertebrae can start touching each other. This is really painful and the whole back is no longer supported. Here again, surgery is the only option and discs are replaced with artificial ones or the vertebrae are fixed together through fusion or metal bars.

8.2. Preventing osteoarthritis and disc degeneration

Regular physical exercise is the only known way to delay osteoarthritis and helps keep the spinal discs healthy as we all have our own hereditary predispositions. Indeed more exercise can increase the creation of blood vessels or maintain a healthy blood flow near the discs.

As said above, cartilage tissue tends to wear off over time. Therefore activities where the joints (and therefore cartilages) are widely solicited tend to lead to osteoarthritis over time. This is why skiers and joggers tend to get knee/back problems and why tennis can lead to elbow issues.

Specifically for spinal discs, good posturing and careful manipulation of heavy weights are to be recommended.

I will get into back issues further, but it is clear that stronger back muscles and abdominal muscles help protect the spinal discs (and thus the whole back) as they will be able to keep the back steadier. They are also able to offset up to a certain point the effect of any sudden unwanted move in the back.

Smoking increases the risks of disc generation and cartilage damage as atherosclerosis and the vasoconstriction provoked by nicotine will reduce even more the blood flow to these tissues which are already fragile by nature (lack of direct blood supply).

Chapter 9: Ligaments

Ligaments are the fibrous tissues that connect *bones* to other bones. They should not be confused with tendons which connect *muscles* to bones.

Ligaments are made of collagen based tissues. They are therefore elastic, but they cannot retain their original shape if stretched for too long. This is why dislocated joints must be put back together as quickly as possible by medical professionals.

Broken ligaments can lead to joint instability. Since joint instability can lead to osteoarthritis, broken ligaments have to be fixed. Sometimes this may require surgery if the ligament is totally torn or far from where it should be.

9.1. Preventing ligament tears in articulations

Ligament fibers are a very strong tissue which can support a lot of tension, but only if the tension goes through the ligaments (i.e. the force is absolutely parallel to the fibers). This is why an arm will not "fall" or dislocate if one is carrying a suitcase. However the ligaments are fragile if the force is not parallel. This is why there are so many injuries in sports such as soccer or skiing where the forces are never totally parallel to the ligaments.

As in other cases, building the muscles around the articulation is the best way to protect the articulations as the muscle can, to a certain degree, offset the force which is going against the ligament. As with the bones, pressure/tension such as those provided by lifting weights can also help reinforce ligaments.

There is not much more to add on ligaments so this is a short chapter. Yayyyy!

Chapter 10: Muscles

Muscles are the soft, fiber like tissues in the body. Muscle cells contain certain protein filaments which enable the contraction of the muscle by a change in the length (and shape) of the cell.

There several types of muscle, but in a nutshell there are 1) the hearts' muscle, 2) the smooth muscles and 3) the skeletal muscles.

The hearts' muscle cells have been discussed in the chapter of the heart and will not be discussed further.

The smooth muscles are also called "involuntary muscles" and are those which are not controlled by the conscious and which are found within organs and structures such as the intestines, the esophagus or the blood vessels. These muscles are controlled by the autonomic nervous system.

The skeletal muscles are those which we usually think of when talking about muscles. They are anchored to the bones though tendons, and enable movement.

We're going to focus on the skeletal muscles here.

10.1. The skeletal muscles

The skeletal muscles are divided into two big groups of fibers: Type I and Type II.

Type I fibers are the "slow" fibers which are used to sustain aerobic activity using fats or carbohydrates as fuel. They require a lot of oxygen and blood.

Type II fibers are the "quick" fibers which are used in the frame of very short and intense anaerobic activity, i.e. they do not have a high oxygen consumption. However, they can only be used for short periods of time before fatigue.

It is the combination of both which enable the body to engage in both short term bursts of activity while also being able to cope with longer periods of activity.

As muscle cells contain protein fibers, the consumption of protein will go in first priority to create muscle cells. This is why athletes (and not only bodybuilders) need high protein intakes.

Protein will only be used as a source of energy in the body if the need for protein by the muscles has been met or if there are no other sources of energy. In this case, the body will convert some of the muscle tissue into fat and the muscle will go through the condition known as atrophy.

While atrophy is a normal condition as one ages, regular exercise can offset a big chunk of it. As said in the chapter on bones, since there is a relation in between muscle mass and bone density, muscle atrophy can be a symptom of a case of osteoporosis.

Also, and as said before, skeletal muscles, can help protect joints (ligaments, cartilage tissue) as their contraction may help offset an involuntary force whose nature could lead to damaging the joint.

Furthermore, as muscles consume a lot of oxygen and blood, the increase in muscle mass due to regular exercise will lead to a growth of new blood vessels which will therefore increase the total blood supply to that region of the body. In some cases, like for cartilages or spinal discs, this increase in blood supply can improve the healing processes.

Chapter 11: Tendons

Tendons are the fibrous tissue which connect the muscles to the bones. As ligaments, tendons are made from collagen fibers.

Tendons are more stretchable/elastic than ligaments, which is why most injuries are related to ligaments and not to tendons. Furthermore tendons resemble to bones in the sense that they respond to changes in their use. I.e. bones will respond to greater "weight" by an increase in bone density. In the same way, tendons will see their strength increase if they are solicited by regular physical exercise. It takes much more time for tendons (and ligaments) to reinforce themselves than it will take time to increase the size/strength/mass of a muscle. This is why people who go to the fitness and start lifting heavy weights right away will gain muscle, but will damage their tendons/ligaments. And one knows how difficult it is to heal from a tendonitis (actually one never really fully recovers as the tendon will remain weakened).

Bottom line: lifting "lighter" weights is necessary when one starts/resumes going to the gym. Since tendons/ligaments will take in between 6-18 months to reinforce themselves, going progressively is really key to avoid injuries.

Hmm really a short chapter this one is[57].

With this ends Part II. Let's go on to the dieting part now!

---

[57] Yoda wouldn't have said better.

Lose weight now!

Part 3: How does the body lose weight in real life?

Okay, now that you have understood the basics of the different nutrients and some of the vital functions and essential body organs/tissues, we have all what it takes to understand the mechanisms which lead to changes in body weight. For most people, the focus is on losing body fat[58].

---

[58] Most people are not going to complain of having too much muscle.

Lose weight now!

Chapter 12: How the body loses weight (in real life)

It is extremely important (and easy) to understand how the body loses weight. Once you understand this, you will quickly understand why so many diets are bogus, and so many "fitness machines" are just an outright scam[59].

12.1. The weight losing process

There are just three simple things to understand about this process:

12.1.1. Body weight equation™ (BWE)[60]

It's a simple equation:

Initial body weight + Calorie intake (food+drinks) - Calories spent (body activity +physical exercise) = Final body weight

No surprise here. It's the difference in between the calories we take and those that we spend that leads to changes in weight. It is therefore obvious that one can eat much more and still lose weight if one spends more calories than what one intakes.

For example, it's well known that top swimmers can have *daily* kilo calorie intakes of more than 10'000 when preparing competitions. This compares with average recommended daily kilo calorie intakes of 2'000 to 3'000 for men and 1'800 to 2'300 for women.

---

[59] Bernie Madoff did not get it right. If he had been in the dieting business he would have made millions selling lies without ever risking jail.
[60] Putting a TM and an acronym really makes the thing look pro, huh?

This is why no serious weight loss can occur without both a change in nutrition *and* a change in lifestyle. The best way to spend calories is doing the *right* physical exercises. This will be discussed later in greater depth.

Durable changes in body weight require a durable difference in between the calories taken and the calories spent. Here again, don't thing about getting to your new physique overnight. It's a process, a journey. It's an endless marathon. Not a sprint.

12.1.2. Body calorie source order

When the body needs energy, it will generate energy (calories used) by using the different nutrients in the following invariable order:

1. Simple Carbohydrates (blood sugar),
2. Complex carbohydrates (glycogen),
3. Lipids,
4. Proteins.

Therefore, since lipids are basically the last energy source to be used, one has to use the carbohydrates available in the body *before* the body starts converting them into energy. This is why short duration or brisk exercises will *never* be able to burn fat.

12.1.3. Body fat locations

When the body starts burning fat, i.e. converting fats into calories, it will choose from which area (of the body) it will take the fats from. We are all different. For some persons, the body will use first the fat in the arms, then in the thighs, then in the buttocks, before using the fat in the belly. For other people the body may start first with the buttocks and then the arm. In all cases, the fat from the belly will be lost last as it's the closest location to many of the vital organs, whereas the limbs (arms and legs) are less important as not vital.

Furthermore, the locations where the body will stock fats is different in between men and women. Since the latter have the ability to carry children, their body will stock even more fat (energy source) close to where the fetus will grow, i.e. the belly and hips.

The TV ads promoting all these abdominal machines as a way to lose weight and get a 6-pack are simply totally false. If nutrition isn't good, one will still get fat despite doing abs the whole day long. Furthermore, in the case that there *were* weight loss, the body will take the fat first from the limps, not the belly (abs).

12.2. Why most diets are not only ineffective, but unhealthy

If diets were not effective, they would just be a waste of money. What makes diets bad is that they are outright unhealthy. There are several reasons for this

12.2.1. Imbalance in nutrients

Many diets will lead to an imbalance in the nutrients taken. While short term the body can live with a surplus or a deficit of certain nutrients, longer tem (i.e. after 15 days) negative consequences will appear. Often they start to show up with symptoms such as fatigue, difficulty to concentrate or focus, irritability. If kept over longer periods of time, severe medical conditions can develop.

12.2.2. Loss of self-esteem

As restrictive diets are not natural, the body will react and one will develop physiological needs which can lead to psychological "cravings". After a while these cravings for food will often lead to "binge eating" or the resumption of earlier eating habits. This is bad because often this will entail eating a lot of unhealthy food. More importantly, once the binge eating is over, one feels ashamed of one's self.

We will start thinking things like "I'm no good, I don't have the will to change my diet" or "I should not have started this diet, I knew that I cannot discipline myself. I always knew I was a loser".

Such thinking just lowers self-esteem and will create a vicious circle where the loss of self-esteem will lead to a loss of confidence. The loss of confidence will lead to a loss in determination to change. And you will return to the "old you". But in worse, since this "old you" will have even less confidence than you had at the beginning. This is why loss of self-esteem and confidence not only leads to poor physical health but also to poor psychological health with conditions such as anxiety, depression (or manic depression), etc. Such conditions can lead to poor sleeping patterns, nervous system disorders, etc. And forget about getting a better physique if you are in depression.

The question of loss of self-esteem is so important that I cannot stress it enough. This is why people who fail one diet often will fail the next diets. And it's because that they have such low self-esteem and such low levels of confidence that they become credulous and believe the next "miracle dieting method".

Lastly, self-esteem and loss confidence also have an effect on social life as well as the private life. This can put couples at risk. And if you're single, you can totally forget about getting someone in such a state of mind.

This is why the Smart Diet™ is good. It does not create these unbearable pressures which will lead to failure. It just follows your rhythm. More on that later.

Chapter 13: Water retention

Excess fats are of course the main reason for overweight. However water retention can be another source of excess weight. This is why I would like to touch on this subject.

13.1. What is water retention?

The body is mainly composed of water. The systems to maintain fluid levels at constant levels are complex and involve the use of hormones. The kidney is the well-known organ that will excrete excess liquids in the form of urine.

Water retention is the abnormal accumulation of water (fluid) in the circulatory system or within certain tissues or cavities of the body. Don't forget that water is found inside and outside the cells. It is found in blood. It is also found in tissues, organs, muscles and bones!

At the cellular level, the smallest blood vessels (i.e. the capillaries) are those where exchanges of nutrients will occur. Remember that the capillary vessels have a permeability which enables these exchanges in between the blood and the cells.

Water retention can occur if the capillaries, become too "leaky" and some excess fluid ends up in the space in between cells. Since not all the excess liquid is able to re-enter the capillary, fluid starts to accumulate in the tissues. It is the accumulation of these fluids in certain tissues that we call "water retention" and that can be visible due to the swelling of the tissues. Due to gravity the swelling of tissues (water retention) often occurs in legs, ankles, feet or the abdomen.

Water retention is a medical condition and you should consult a doctor if you have (or suspect you have) this condition.

13.2. Causes of water retention

There are several causes or factors which can lead to water retention.

13.2.1. Capillary "leakage"

As said above, this is the condition where too much fluid is able to leave the capillary, thus leading to an accumulation in the tissues. There can be different causes for capillary leakage and I will not go in detail in all of them. However one cause of such leakage is a deficiency in molecules known as "flavonoids" that impact the permeability of the capillaries.

Flavonoids can be found in citrus fruits (grapefruit, lemon, orange, and lime), tea, wine and dark chocolate (not milk chocolate). Who said that healthy food was not tasty?

In the case of capillary leakage, diuretic drugs (i.e. medicines that favor liquid removal by the kidneys) is not advised as it can be dangerous. Indeed they will tend to drain water from the blood (blood dehydration), while at the same time fluid will remain in the tissues or even increase.

13.2.2. Heart and/or lung failures

The pumping force of the heart should help keep a normal pressure within blood vessels. However in the case of heart or lung failure, this pressure can change thus leading to massive water retention. In this case, diuretics are a good treatment.

13.2.3. Protein deficiency

Protein attracts water and therefore plays an important role in water balance. In the case of severe protein deficiencies the blood may not have enough protein to attract the water from the tissues back into the capillaries. This is the reason why people who have starving often have an enlarged abdomen: the lack of protein leads to insufficient water getting back into the blood stream, thus accumulating in the abdomen.

13.2.4. Histamines

Histamines are very important molecules which are released when there is a body inflammation. They tend to widen the capillaries thus making them more "leaky". In a normal body, this is to enable white blood cells to get out of the blood stream and go to the site of the inflammation more quickly. Of course, unless the inflammation is chronic, there is no long-term water retention.

13.2.5. Kidney failures

As the kidney is the main organ involved in removing water, any kidney failure or disease will lead to water retention. The kidney is a very complex organ so I will not get into further detail here. If you want to learn more on the subject, check out the internet, because even your traditional medical generalist will be lost on the subject of kidneys.

13.2.6. Pregnancy

Late stage pregnancy can cause temporary water retention as the weight of the uterus on the major veins of the pelvis will lead to more fluid leaving the capillaries. Most of the time, once the baby is delivered by DHL (or Fedex or UPS[61]) this condition disappears. If not, a medical doctor should be consulted.

---

[61] It's a trap! Just to see if you were still concentrated. However if you do believe that babies are delivered by DHL or another of those delivery companies, please ask one of your parents to have with you that serious discussion about bees, grains, flowers and babies.

13.2.7. Premenstrual water retention

This is a common phenomenon associated with the menstrual cycle. It is a temporary condition but it can be noticeable by an uncomfortable enlargement of the breasts and/or breast tenderness. This can be due to hormone imbalances during this period but can be accentuated by the lack of certain nutrients such as vitamins B1, B5 and B6 or magnesium. The dietary sources for these nutrients will be mentioned further in the book.

13.2.8. Medicines

Certain medical drugs can lead to water retention. These include estrogen containing drugs such as those used in hormone replacement therapies. Combined oral contraceptive (birth control pills) may in *some* cases increase water retention, however most studies do not link taking the pill to any significant weight gains.

Beta-blockers which are used in the case of heart arrhythmias may also lead to water retention. Analgesics in high doses can lead to the same condition.

13.3. Prevention and treatment of water retention

In the case where there is a significant water retention problem, and that its source isn't the leaky capillaries, diuretics can be a powerful treatment (but only under the strict guidance and supervision of a medical doctor).

However, in the cases which are not significant enough to justify diuretics or simply to prevent water retention there are several things you can do.

13.3.1. Nutrition

As said above, increasing the consumption of "flavonoids" will impact favorably the permeability of the capillaries and can reduce leakage. The consumption of citrus fruits (grapefruit, lemon, orange, lime), tea, wine and dark chocolate (not milk chocolate) can help restore a good balance in the body.

Also as said above, for women the consumption of vitamins B1, B5 and B6 or magnesium is also helpful during their menstrual cycle.

Another easy was to reduce water retention is to reduce the consumption of salt since salt favors water retention.

Finally since the body will tend to stock water to avoid "shortages", the more one drinks (on a regular basis) the less the body will feel the need to build water reserves. So if you want to lose your "love handles" which is a place with often a lot of water, drink more water more regularly. If you're an adult, you should be drinking about 2.5 liters of water[62] per day in normal circumstances. Of course, you will need much more when it's hot or when you do physical exercise.

13.3.2. Regular physical exercise

Since water retention is accentuated by gravity, regular exercise can help by moving the blood around faster. Having more "blood movement" will avoid blood to pool in the leg veins, thus creating pressures on the capillaries which will increase leakage, thus water retention.

Another important benefit of physical exercises is their role in the lymphatic system. So let's talk briefly about the lymphatic system. The lymphatic system is basically the "sewer system" of the body. It is an "open system" which has several functions including removing interstitial fluids from tissues (i.e. the fluids in between cells) and transporting white blood cells from the bones to the lymph nodes

---

[62] It's of course water that I'm talking about since it's well known that alcohol dehydrates.

where they are stocked. The first function is of course the one related to water retention.

Unlike the circulatory system which has the heart as pumping organ, there is no dedicated organ to pump the lymph which is the name of the liquid substance running through the lymphatic vessels. Therefore in the body of a person who does not do regular exercise, the fluids which are absorbed by the lymphatic vessels will just stay there since there is no "pump" to move the fluids out of the way.

Muscles do play the role of pump for the lymphatic system by pure mechanical pressures on the lymphatic vessels. Physical exercises will lead to the contraction of muscles and an increase of muscle volume. This will pump the lymph from the lymphatic vessels all the way to their final destination which are the subclavian veins (two large veins on both sides of the spine). There the lymph will join in the blood flow and the excess liquids will be removed by the kidney.

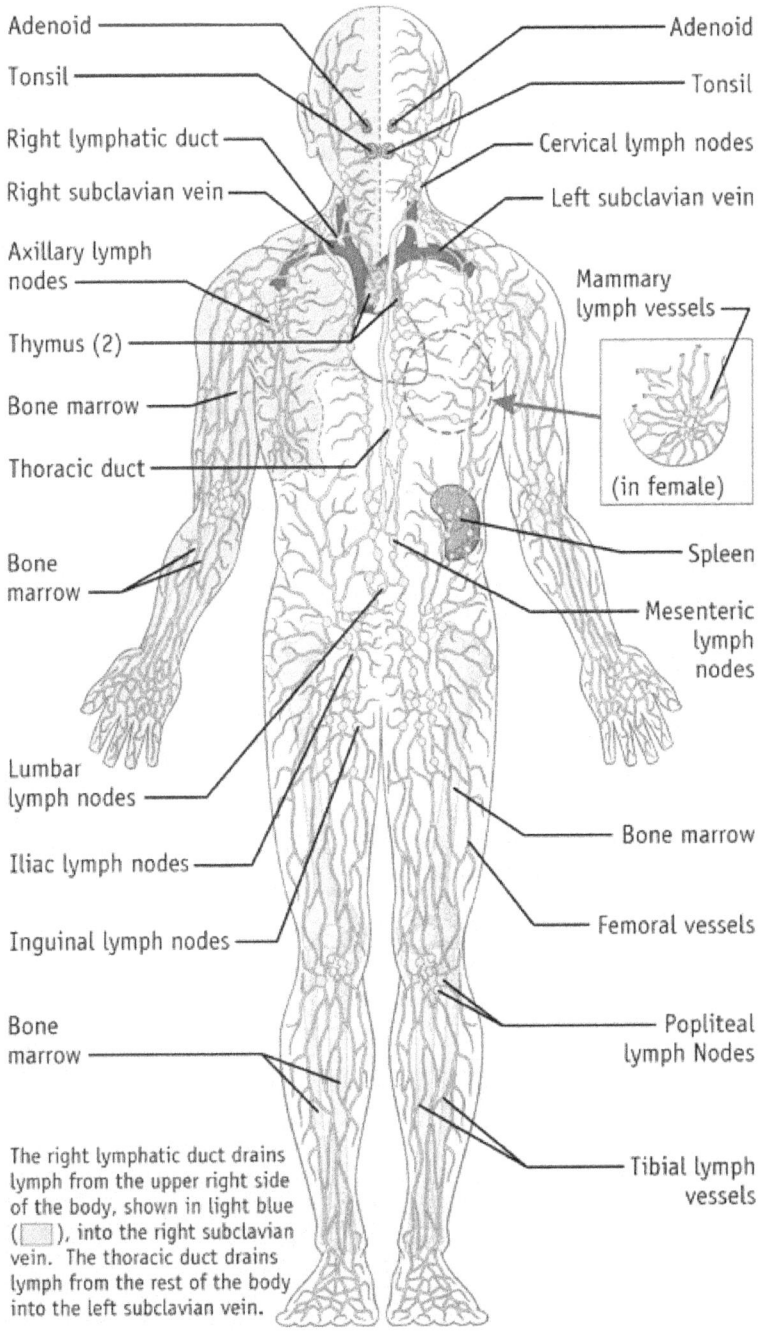

Adenoid — Adenoid
Tonsil — Tonsil
Right lymphatic duct — Cervical lymph nodes
Right subclavian vein — Left subclavian vein
Axillary lymph nodes —
Mammary lymph vessels —
Thymus (2) —
Bone marrow —
Thoracic duct —
(in female)
Bone marrow — Spleen
Mesenteric lymph nodes
Lumbar lymph nodes —
Iliac lymph nodes — Bone marrow
Inguinal lymph nodes — Femoral vessels
Bone marrow — Popliteal lymph Nodes

The right lymphatic duct drains lymph from the upper right side of the body, shown in light blue (☐), into the right subclavian vein. The thoracic duct drains lymph from the rest of the body into the left subclavian vein.

Tibial lymph vessels

Source: Hilmerstudios.com

13.3.3. Posturing

Avoiding to stand up or sit for too long helps move the blood and avoids blood to pool. This is why when traveling in cars, trains, planes, boats, it is important to move your legs and change positions. Raising the legs several times per day may also help improve circulation.

13.3.4. Stockings

For those with water retention issues in lower limps, supporting stalkings can help. Overweight persons are more vulnerable to water retention. But in the case that an overweight person starts to change his/her nutrition and lifestyle, stockings may eventually no longer be needed.

13.3.5. Massages

Since the lymphatic system does not have a pump, simple massages can help. You just need to apply pressure with the hands and always go in direction of the heart (since the subclavian veins are close to the heart). Be sure to apply enough pressure, a lymphatic massage has to be firm, it's not about caressing[63].

---

[63] You can do that after!

Part 4: Why the well known diets don't work in real life

Now that we know how the body and the nutrients work, now that we know what makes the body lose weight, let's analyze some of the well-known diets, and see why they simply cannot work over the long-run and why, much to the opposite, they can lead to health problems.

This is the part where we are going to tear down the myths and lies of some of these much hyped and marketed diets.

For sake of simplicity of reading, the analysis of the different diets will follow a similar structure.

Lose weight now!

Chapter 14: The main categories of diets

There are basically four categories of diets. Most known diets fall within one of these categories.

These categories are:

1) Low fat diets,
2) Low carbohydrate diets,
3) Low calorie diets,
4) Very low calorie diets.

14.1. Low fat diets

Low fat diets are those that include little fat intake. Calorie consumption is reduced because less fat is consumed. While diets with higher intakes of vegetables and fruits, less diary products and less red meat have been associated with lower heart diseases, their effectiveness as far as long lasting weight loss is not apparent. Indeed, as we have seen in chapter 2, lipids are essential to life. No fat, no life. Therefore these low fat diets cannot be applied for a long time without starting to create health problems.

14.2. Low carbohydrate diets (low carb diets)

Low carb diets are generally high in protein and fats. They restrict carbohydrate intake. Foods with high carbohydrates (carbs) such as pasta or bread are replaced with foods having higher percentages of proteins or fats (meats, eggs, cheese). Fruits and vegetables are also often included. The proponents of low carb diets think that it's an easier way to lose weight.

Low carb diets will usually restrict carbs to less than 20% of the total caloric intake. In some cases they can be used to manage certain health conditions such as diabetes, epilepsy or polycystic ovarian syndrome.[64] However, in these cases this type of diet must be done under strict medical supervision.

Of course, we all know that too much simple carbs (e.g. sugars) can lead to fat creation, however the idea that the body can replace much of its carbs by fats, is far from being a positive medical certainty. While the body can adapt to a low carb diet over time, there will be issues of fatigue and lack of dynamism. Since simple carbs are used in the frame of short/intense physical activities (when the body performs in an anaerobic mode), people following low carb diets will have worse performances than those with normal eating habits. Low carb diets can also lead to hypoglycemia in certain cases.

Moreover, we know that many fats are not healthy, so it's not easy to get enough energy for the body by eating fats while at the same time trying to avoid the bad fats. In fact the "typical" low carb meal with a steak of red meat and some vegetables can be a real killer meal with low nutritional value (in the sense that not only eating regularly red meat will end up shortening your life expectancy, but the amount of nutrients found in that kind of meal can be low). And we know today that medicine recommends limiting red meat to once a week. In some cases, low carb advocates reduce the intake of fruits and vegetables, thus depriving the body of important sources of nutrients.

In addition, low carb diets can lead to a condition known as ketosis. When the body does not have enough glucose in the blood, the pancreas will secrete a hormone, glucagon, that will stimulate the liver to convert stored glycogen into blood and release it in the blood. When this is not enough, fatty acids are converted into molecules known as ketones which the brain can use as energy source. The problem is that with low carb diets and the more important presence of ketones in the blood (hyperketonemia), there are risk of acidosis, i.e. a change in the acidity of the blood. Extreme levels of acidosis can lead to death. Less extreme side effects

---

[64] In some cases, it was found that a high fat low carb diet helps women with polycystic ovary syndrome. Indeed this condition is characterized by insulin resistance which will therefore tend to convert estrogen into testosterone. In turn this can increase infertility.

associated to ketosis include: headaches, weakness, dizziness, nausea or stomach aches, bad breath[65], sleep problems, fatigue, etc.

The medical benefits for low carb diets for people without a medical condition remain largely unproven. Some studies have indicated higher medical risks for people following low carb diets. Studies mentioned increased risk in the following areas:

- Increased risk of kidney stone formation (due to the change in acidity of the blood),

- Increased risk of bone loss.

Some studies have noted higher mortality rates among the population following low carb diets. Low carb diets also can lead to symptoms such as fatigue, lack of dynamism, lack of concentration and focus. Constipation is also a well known side-effect of low carb diets due to a lack of fiber intake, a lake of overall food volume intake, etc. Clearly eating a lot red meat or cheese does not help the intestinal transit (i.e. the motivation of the body to go to the bathroom). Of course advocates of the low carb diets will have suggestions to try to avoid some of the negative side-effects of low carb diets by adding or removing parts of the diet or even taking laxatives (!). That becomes an awfully complicated mess to manage with possible side-effects of the "remedies" supposed to deal "initial" side-effects of the low carb diet. I have another suggestion: forget about low carb diets altogether,

Low carb diets have only really been shown to give positive effects over the long term when the objective is to deal with a serious medical condition such as epilepsy (as well as autism and some other neuronal conditions), diabetes, etc. So unless you have a medical condition that justifies a low carb diet, and that your diet has been made by a professional nutritionist and that you diet under the supervision of a medical doctor, forget about low carb diets.

---

[65] This side effect probably is enough to have most people want to stop right away with their low carb diet.

Of course, if someone eats pizza and fast food the whole day and only drinks sodas, any kind of diet will show results. However the benefits of low carb diets over balanced diets are not proven. However some of the health risks of low carb diets are proven.

So which are some of the well known, bogus diets that fall in the category of the low carb category? Unsurprisingly, many known diets are of this type.

14.2.1. Atkins diet

This old diet, which was written in 1958, is based on the idea that burning fat uses more calories than burning carbs. Of course this is wrong, and it's funny to notice that a wrong idea has not prevented the Atkins diet to still be popular today. Although much less since the Atkins Nutritional company filed for Chapter 11 bankruptcy in 2005. The fact that some doctors link the high protein low carb diet to increased heart disease probably didn't help (many doctors now recommend not eating red meat more than once a week).

Like all diets, the Atkins diets came with some kind of plan that is complicated and with contradictions (whether some fats are good or not, which ones to take, which ones to avoid, etc). Bottom line: don't waste your time with this diet.

14.2.2. Paleolithic diet also known as paleo or Stone Age diet

So this is the diet that Kim tried. A friend of hers is also a big fan of this. So how can I write that the paleo is just a waste of time without risking being de-friended until the end of times? Should I try to be diplomatic about the whole thing? Hell no! I'm going to be as direct and as fact driven as usual! Muahahahaha (sadistic mode on).

The paleo diet was popularized in the mid 1970s by a US gastroenterologist, Walter Voegtlin, who had the idea that less carbs would lead to better health. Some advocates of paleo say that a reduced carb intake leads to less insulin responses (as there is less carb intake, the body will produce less insulin), less inflammatory risks[66], and therefore a reduced risk factor for many diseases. They also say that the dieting habits of the "humans" of the Paleolithic period era (i.e. 2.5 million years ago to approx. 10'000 years ago) were based primarily on a low carb diet (meat, fruits and vegetables). They also note that many of the "modern illnesses" affecting today's population (heart diseases, high blood pressure, obesity, etc) did not affect the "hunter gatherers" which lived 25'000 years ago, before the agricultural revolution.

I don't really know how life was 25'000 or 40'000 years ago. Well, probably if you were a guy it was easier pick up a girl because all you had to do is to pull her by her hair and drag her to your cave. And that practice may even have been considered as "socially acceptable"… Unless in reality it was the other way around… We're not sure…

In any case, I don't know how anybody in his right mind could want to take lifestyle habits from the Paleolithic era to today's world. Which woman would switch her bikini shave from "Brazilian wax style" to "Paleolithic style", i.e. ten centimeter hair everywhere, from head to toe (any maybe longer under the armpits)? Which guy would like to get a deodorant with the vintage "Paleolithic scent", i.e. the smell you get after spending 10 years without a shower and sleeping on mud? Who would exchange his/her bed for a humid cavern? You get the point.

From a health perspective, one should also remember that maybe one of the reasons that our paleo ancestors did not have some of our modern illnesses was that they did not live long enough to get them. I mean getting to your thirties at that time was already quite a feat. Maybe another reason they did not have some of those illnesses is that they spent more time doing physical activities (they were obliged to) than most people today. They also didn't have the pollution and stress we have today. Probably they were not as obese due to the fact that there were periods of hunger and starvation due

---

[66] As seen before, inflammatory reactions can be high not only due to carbs but also to saturated fatty acids.

to poor weather conditions. But maybe they did in fact already suffer some of our "modern" diseases. Science did prove that even 20'000 years ago, our ancestors starting eating cereals (this comes from the scientific analysis of teeth coming from skulls dated to the Paleolithic era).

Bottom line: the paleo diet does not have any scientific proof of leading to an over all better health. Some of the modern illnesses are caused in part by stress, pollution agents, our sedentary lifestyles as well as the junk food we eat. Not by eating cereals. So, Kim, I hope you see why your 200 page book on the cavemen diet was a waste of time (you should have bought a cooking book to learn how to do brownies and pancakes instead!).

14.3. Low calorie diets (low cal diets)

Low calorie diets will usually produce energy deficits of 500-1000 calories per day, therefore reducing weight. Obviously, any diet based on a calorie deficit will induce weight loss. And of course, any fat reduction will decrease health risk. However, this diet has many negative side effects such as muscle mass loss and a reduction of bone density since the body will have to offset the calorie deficit through burning fat as well as other tissues.

The process of catabolism (which means that the body will break elements to produce energy) will involve the production in greater quantities of catabolic hormones such as cortisol which will tend to disrupt protein synthesis. Catabolic hormones also will negatively affect the immune system response. No wonder that some studies found that low calorie diets are associated to higher mortality levels! In other words, these diets kill you slowly.

Furthermore low calorie diets are found to trigger eating disorders such as cravings and binge eating. As mentioned in section 12.2.2. such disorders affect the self-esteem and reduce even more the motivation to eat healthy.

Low calorie diets also may lead to ovulatory dysfunctions and increased infertility for women. For pregnant women, these diets put greater health risk on their baby. If this weren't enough, low calorie diets also lead to a condition of fatigue and loss of concentration, which can lead those who follow such a diet to intake fast sugars (often junk food sweets or drinks) or high caffeine intakes (through coffee, Red bull or other drinks). In turn this will lead to other negative side effects.

Low calorie diets are also very unhealthy for children who need a lot of energy and healthy food to grow up. And I'm not talking only about size. I'm also taking about brain/nervous system health as well as a healthy hormonal system.

So which are some of the well known diets which fall in the category of the unhealthy low calorie category? You well be surprised to see that many well known diets fall in this category.

14.3.1. Weight Watchers diet

The current plan offered in the US has as objective to create a deficit in terms of calories per day, thus forcing the body to burn fat to offset the calorie deficit.

This diet uses a system of "points" to help participants select what foods they eat and in which quantities.

Other than being a very popular unhealthy diet, the Weight Watcher diet is complicated. Who the f*%k wants to have to go through formulas such as those before eating?

$$PointsPlus = max\left\{ round\left(\frac{(16 \cdot protein) + (19 \cdot carbohydrates) + (45 \cdot fat) - (14 \cdot fiber)}{175} \right), 0 \right\}$$

$$PointsPlus = max\left\{ round\left(\frac{protein}{10.9375} + \frac{carbohydrates}{9.2105} + \frac{fat}{3.8889} - \frac{fiber}{12.5} \right), 0 \right\}$$

If I'm hungry, I want to eat right away without having to solve some silly mathematical equations. I don't know about you, but I tell you, you're never gonna see my white ass doing this kind of stuff anytime soon. Do note that I skipped the different coefficients taken for different ages, sex[67], etc. So the whole diet is really confusing.

Also, who the f%*k wants to pay cash to be member of a "club of the fat people" and go through some kind of lame and stultifying[68] group therapy? Who wants to pay money to have the "privilege" to be part of a club of the losers? If you want to eat healthy and lose weight, the resolve has to come from within you, not from someone else. If you believe the opposite, go live in Disneyland because that's where you belong.

To me, it's unbelievable that Weight Watcher still exists. I guess it's like a sect that gets so much money from its gullible members that it's able to attract every day new losers to its club. As Einstein said "Human silliness and the universe are infinite, although I'm not sure of the latter[69]".

14.3.2. Nutrisystems diet

Same ideas as Weight Watchers with costs related to the programs and some kind of community. However, unlike J.R.R. Tolkien's "Fellowship of the Ring", it's a "fellowship of the people not able to look good in a bikini or in swimming trunks". Yeah, they do promote physical exercise, like 10 minutes of moderate intensity activity per day. Are you kidding me? Ten minutes a day?

---

[67] In this context, I'm talking about gender. Weight watchers do not go as far as to impose to their members that they resolve mathematical equations while getting laid or laying some pipe.

[68] Stultifying means to dumb down. Yaay! I learned a word! Thanks internet.

[69] We know today that the universe is not infinite but "only" 80bn light years across. String theory also suggests that we are in a multiverse with possibly an infinite number of "bubble" type universes, floating in some kind of cosmic "soda".

If you think that 10 minutes of moderate exercise is going to help reduce fat, you are definitely in for some serious disappointment in life. So here is some more shocking truth for you: Justin Bieber doesn't know how to sing. And the tooth fairy doesn't exist either, get over it.

14.3.3. Other diets

The world is never short of people wanting to try to make money by selling the "new" and "hot" diet method. So there are many diets within the low calorie category. Other names include the Body for Life diet, the Hacker's diet, etc. I'm not going to waste more time on low calorie diets, because I hope you understand by now how bad they are for your health. If you didn't, please read this whole section again. If that doesn't work, I'm afraid there is no hope for you and your intelligence deprived brain... your only hope is to get into politics where intellectually challenged persons are not only accepted, but are even able to thrive.

14.4. Very low calorie diets (very low cal diets)

Very low calorie diets are a more extreme variant of the low calorie diet. They tend to maintain protein intake but reduce the calories from fats and carbs. Very low carb diets are basically a form of starvation and are therefore not recommended. They are down right dangerous and besides the loss of many human tissues, they will have many secondary effects.

This is why very low calorie diets are often short in terms or duration and used in the frame of a medical condition. As such these diets are followed under the strict supervision of a medical doctor.

Some "religious" traditions involve extended periods of starvation. I'm not going to go into detail on this, however I will just mention that those who follow (followed) them end up dead or with serious medical conditions. In other words, it's totally stupid and against nature/life.

14.5. Other types of diets

14.5.1. Vegetarianism

Vegetarianism is not a diet per say as it does not focus on weight loss or healthy eating. It does not focus on the mix of protein, lipids, carbs and minerals. Instead it only focuses on what not to eat (basically it excludes meats and foods derived from animals).

Vegetarianism has no scientific background and is only motivated by various religious beliefs or other beliefs such as animal rights, etc[70].

Vegetarianism has several varieties:

- The ovo-vegetarian diet includes eggs but not diary products,

- The lacto-vegetarian diet includes diary products but not eggs,

- The ovo-lacto vegetarian diet includes diary products and eggs,

- The vegan diet (or strictly vegetarian diet) excludes all animal products including eggs, diary, honey, etc.

Okay now this is my book, right? And I said I was going to be direct and straight-to-your-face, right? So enough with politically correct stuff: vegetarianism is plain bullshit and down right stupid. There you go. Humans are omnivores (check out your biology class notes if you have any kind of doubt) and there is no need for any kind of restriction on eating food derived from animals.

Humans are not herbivores and we cannot spend 8 hours[71] a day eating salad and stuff to get the calories we need.

---

70 It's also trendy in places where intelligence is clearly not a socially important criteria. The show business industry is such a place.
71 True fact: cows actually spend up to 8 hours per day eating in order to get their calories.

From a nutritional point of view, vegetarianism is an unhealthy and unbalanced diet as one does not get the quality and quantity of the necessary nutrients for our body. Several types of proteins are for example only found in meat, and of course in greater quantity than in any kind of vegetable or grain.

Another example is DHA (Docosahexaenoic acid) which is the omega 3 fatty acid that is a primary component of the human brain, skin, sperm, retina, etc. DHA is found in maternal milk or fish oil. Since adults cannot breast feed from their mother anymore, and that guys cannot breast feed from their girlfriend/wife on a daily basis, eating fish or taking DHA/fish oil pills are the only options available.

Insufficient DHA is linked to things like Alzheimer, cancer, retina disorders, etc. Pregnant women without enough DHA intake put the health of the fetus at risk. It has been shown that vegetarian diets typically contain insufficient levels of DHA, putting these persons at risk.

I'm not going to go any further because you get the point. Vegetarianism is stupid and dangerous for your health. If you are a vegan, change your diet if you still have some intelligence left in your DHA deprived brain. Nevertheless if you still think that vegetarianism is okay, stop reading this book and go get yourself a therapist.

14.5.2. Detox diets

Detoxification diets (detox diets) are not diets focused on weight loss. They come from the idea that once in a while, one should engage in certain "eating practices" in order to "purify" the body from toxins and other harmful substances which it produces. While the idea was popular in ancient Egypt and Greece, this idea has fallen out of favor with modern medicine.

Detox diets often include some form of fasting and are often high on fibers. They will also tend to include herbs, celery and other juicy, low calorie vegetables. Of course, fasting is dangerous and fibers are to be including in any healthy diet. So detox diets are at the best some kind of scam with little negative side effects if they are limited to the ingestion of harmless substances taken in homeopathic quantities.

For most people a "detox diet" is what they will do when they have a hangover[72] after having drunk too much vodka or other cocktails at a nightclub, i.e. fruit juices, water, vegetables and light food. As vegetarianism, detox diets often find fans among those in the show business industry.

14.5.3. Intermittent fasting

Intermittent fasting, is the "new" kid on the block as far as diet. Not. Actually the idea of fasting and intermittent fasting is really very old and dates back to probably a few thousand years ago, although at that time, it was either due to religious believes or lack of sufficient food.

Nevertheless, intermittent fasting has been presented as a new way to lose weight, especially popular among hipsters. As said in section 14.4, any diet based on an insufficient intake of calories will have as effect a reduction in fat (and weight) as you are basically starving the body. As said before, in this case the body will start to burn the fats and then the muscles in order to ensure sufficient energy for the vital organs (which, for hipsters, do not include the brain).

So why is intermittent fasting bad?

While weight loss through intermittent fasting is in theory correct, in real life, the fact of fasting one day before eating the next one can lead to eating disorders (binge eating, excessive eating). Medical

---

[72] From a scientific point of view, to recover the best from a hangover you need to drink a lot of water (to hydrate) as well as eat fruits (preferably some of the aciditic fruits such as apples, oranges or lemons) in order to get simple sugars as well as other acids which will help alleviate the symptoms of the hangover.

studies have also seem to show a relationship in between fasting and higher blood pressure which is a big no-no.

Intuitively, it's quite clear to understand that it is better to eat balanced everyday and to have the energy to do physical exercise on a regular basis, rather than fasting one day, not having the energy to engage in physical exercises and then eat junk food the day you are permitted to eat.

The conclusion is, dear reader, quite obvious. Intermittent fasting is just another marketing idea which actually can lead to real health issues. Bottom line: just stay away from it.

14.6. Losing weight: fat loss versus muscle loss

The objective of any healthy diet has as objective the loss of fat (and not getting it back). The objective is certainly not to lose weight by losing water or muscle mass! As muscle is denser and heavier than fat, a healthy nutrition and lifestyle (physical exercises) will actually involve weight losses by burning the fats and some weight gain by the added muscle mass/bone density. Of course the weight loss of the fats burned will be much greater than the weight gained by the added muscle/bone density. ;-)

Losing water, which is often stored around the waist, should also come through an increased consumption of water and physical exercise. Any kind of dehydration or use of diuretics is silly and will only lead to potential health issues (kidney fatigue, etc).

Enough of the BS diets, it's time for the Smart Diet™!

Lose weight now!

Part 5: The Smart Diet™

This is the part of the book where "the rubber meets the road".

After having read part 1 on the nutrients, part 2 on the human body, part 3 on how the body loses weight in life and part 4 on why the well known diets don't work, you are ready to understand the Smart Diet™[73].

You will see that there is no "voodoo black magic" and that it's all about common sense. How reassuring.

---

[73] I can't get enough of putting the trademark symbol everywhere. It makes me feel important.

Lose weight now!

Chapter 15: The basics of the Smart Diet™

The Smart Diet is awfully simple to understand, especially after having read the previous chapters.

The Smart Diet is based on three postulates based on scientific facts.

15.1. The three postulates of the Smart Diet

There are just three simple things to understand about this diet. Yups, you got it right, only three simple things, no complicated formulas or hog wash.

---

1. The body needs a balanced diet

The body needs proteins, fats, carbohydrates as well as vitamins and minerals to function properly. Any prolonged period of imbalance will create stress on certain body organs/functions which will inevitably lead to one or several medical conditions.

---

2. Initial body weight + Calorie intake - Calories spent = Final body weight

This is the Body weight equation mentioned in chapter 12. It's obvious that focusing on calorie intake only will not work. Especially as over time the metabolism of the body slows and the calories spent tend to decrease as people become more and more sedentary.

One has therefore to focus on the difference in between calorie intake and calories spent.

3. It's a life style. Not a diet!

The Smart Diet is not a diet, it's a life style. It's not something that you do for two or three months. It's a way of living that you adapt in order to be and stay healthy. Since it's something that is meant to be done as long as possible, it has to be adapted to you. Forget diets that will create cravings that will lead to binge eating episodes followed by loss of self esteem and a negative psychological state of mind.

15.2. What are the implications of the three postulates of the Smart Diet?

The **postulate 1** means that you should eat everything, including lipids (fats) and carbohydrates (sugar). There is no limitation of what you should eat as long as its mostly unsaturated fatty acids and complex carbs. Of course one has to increase the intake of "good quality" nutrients and reduce the intake of "bad quality" nutrients.

Note that I say "reduce" the intake of "bad quality nutrients" and not "avoid" them. Indeed **postulate 3** says that the Smart Diet is a life style and not a short term diet plan. We all have cravings for certain types of "junk food". It's normal, we're only human. The idea is that while we put an emphasis on "good nutrients", we also have "cheat meals" which contain some of the "bad quality stuff". These cheat meals are important as they avoid creating frustrations and cravings that lead to binge eating and loss of self-esteem. Cheat meals are important as they enable to keep the motivation high to focus on the "good nutrients". The idea is that if you eat "quality food" 90% of the time, and "junky stuff" 10% of the time, you will be improving your diet overall. And by eating once in a while "junky stuff", you will be remain motivated to eat healthy 90% of the time while avoiding any frustrations building up. I will discuss the nature and frequency of the cheat meals in chapter 16.2.

Postulate 2, only focuses on the difference in between calorie intake and calories spent. There is therefore no limit as far as how much you should eat (as long as its "quality foods"). If you do a lot of physical exercise you can of course eat much more than if you do little physical activity.

15.3. In-depth look at postulate #1: "The body needs a balanced diet, i.e. eat everything!"

Postulate 1 says that you should eat everything, while of course focusing on "good quality" nutrients and limiting the intake of "poor quality" nutrients to a few "cheat meals".

Depending on the amount of weight that you would like to lose, you should reduce the intake of certain foods and limit them to your cheat meals. So basically, it's not about what to eat or what not to eat. It's about how much of it you eat

So let's see what is the "good quality" food that you should be eating most of the time and what is the "poor quality" food that you should only be eating as part of a "cheat meal". The frequency of the cheat meals will be discussed further.

15.3.1. Good quality foods and drinks

Below is a short, non exhaustive list of quality foods and drinks. By good quality foods I mean those foods/meals prepared from, or based on the following:

"Good quality" food	**Comments**
- Fresh vegetables	- Contain many vitamins and minerals as well as antioxidants. Good source of dietary fibers.
- Fresh fruits	- Contain many vitamins and minerals as well as antioxidants. Good source of dietary fibers.
- Non processed white meat (i.e. chicken, turkey, veal)	- Low percentage of fat, high quality proteins.
- Fish, algaes	- Good source of quality protein. A lot of omega-3 and essential fatty acids. Avoid shark, swordfish, which have high mercury content[74]. For the same reason, limit tuna intake to a maximum of 4 cans per week per adult

---

[74] Mercury from natural (volcano) and human (pollution) sources end in fish, with those at the end of the food chain accumulating the most. Mercury in fish is found in the form of methylmercury which can take several days for the body to be eliminated through a process starting with the thyroid glands, the liver and finally the kidneys. This process is not only long but also strains the aforementioned organs. Methylmercury can also accumulate in the brain where it can, if in great enough quantities, lead to several neurological illnesses and pathologies.

- Whole grains (wheat, corn, oats, rice, etc.)	- Good quality carbs. Good source of dietary fibers.
- Olive oil	- High level of monounsaturated fatty acids, polyphenols (antioxidants). Olive oil's fatty acids are also thought to help prevent certain reactions which can lead to Alzheimer's disease.
- Sweet potatoes	- Good quality carbs. Good source of dietary fibers.
- Unsalted nuts, almonds, etc.	- Contain many vitamins and minerals and unsaturated fatty acids.
- Diary products (yogurts, etc.)	- Contain many vitamins, proteins and minerals.
"Good quality" drinks	**Comments**
- Mineral water	- There is no better drink to hydrate the body.
- Green tea, red tea (rooibos)	- High content of antioxidants (polyphenols and flavonoids).
- Red wine	- High content of antioxidants (but avoid taking more than 1 glass per day).
- Milk	- Contains many vitamins, proteins and minerals.

You can eat as much of these foods as you want (within reason of course).

15.3.2. "Poor quality" foods

Below is a short, non exhaustive list of "poor quality" foods and drinks. By "poor quality" foods I mean those foods/meals prepared from, or based on the following:

"Poor quality" food	**Comments**
- Processed foods (frozen foods, ready to eat foods, and basically all industrially produced foods whether sweet or salty)	- They contain many low quality carbs (simple sugars) and often a lot of saturated fats, as well as transfats. This is done by the food companies to give their products "good" taste at a cheap cost. Often low nutritional values for minerals and vitamins. Often high levels of salt.
- Fast food restaurants' meals	- Same as above.
- Fried stuff (French fries, fried vegetables, etc.)	- Many saturated fatty acids and transfats. High salt content.
- Chips	- Many saturated fatty acids and transfats, Low quality carbs. High salt content.
- Sausages, bacon, and other red meat derived products	- High levels of saturated fats and transfats. High salt content.
- Red meat	- Despite the presence of iron, red meat contains a lot of undesirable saturated fats.

- Ice cream, industrial cookies, salty snacks, etc.	- Low quality carbs, high levels of salt and saturated fats.
"Poor quality" drinks	**Comments**
- Alcohol	- Dehydrates the body and has intoxication effects. Alcohol is also a strong carcinogen[75]. See section 15.3.3. below.
- Sodas	- High content of simple sugars. Lots of artificial colorants and/or taste enhancers, some of which are not healthy on the long run[76].
- Energy drinks	- High levels of simple sugars as well as stimulants which can lead to life threatening heart tachycardia (see section 5.3.2.). Also contain high levels of artificial colorants and/or taste enhancers.

These foods are basically unhealthy and harmful over the long term. Remember that while 5-10% of cancers are due to genetic factors, 90-95% of cancers are due to environmental factors:

- Tobacco: 25-30%,
- Obesity: 30-35%,
- Infections: 15-20%,
- Radiations: 0-10%.

---

[75] A carcinogen is a substance or radiation which is directly involved in causing cancer.
[76] Make no mistake. Artificial colorants and flavor enhancers, preservatives and other substances cannot be healthy. At the very best they do no harm.

This means that approximately one third of cancers are related to the consequences of the accumulation of saturated fatty acids in the body as well as the consequences of the high inflammatory states which follow.

This is why the foods and drinks above should only eaten them as part of a "cheat meal". See chapter 16.2.

15.3.3. Foods which can be "ok" or harmful depending on how much you eat of them

Below is a short table of certain foods which can be "okay" if taken in small quantities or not regularly, but which can be harmful when consumed in bigger quantities or on a regular basis.

Foods which can be "ok" or harmful depending on consumption"	Comments
- Cakes, cookies, doughnuts and other backed sweet foods (whether home made or industrially produced)	- They include many low quality carbs (simple sugars). Those prepared industrially or in fast foods often include a lot of saturated fats, transfats and salt.
- Potatoes (regular potatoes: not the sweet ones)	- Include relatively short chains of carbohydrates.
- Eggs	- High cholesterol levels in egg yolks. Excess egg consumption increases cardiovascular risks and may induce liver fatigue.
- Cheese	- Can contain minerals and proteins but also contain a lot of saturated fats.

These foods are basically okay in consumed in "reasonable quantities" and if not eaten "all the time". If you are not able to be reasonable then you should consider these foods as "cheat meals" (see chapter 16.2).

15.3.4. A few words about alcohol

Alcohol has longed been consumed by man due to its intoxication properties including a decrease in desinhibition. As all guys know "drunk girls can't say no" which increases the odds of scoring. The opposite unfortunately doesn't work as girls (and guys) know "drunk boys can't stay hard" which in this case puts the odds of scoring to basically zero.

From a biological point of view, the reason is that alcohol will inhibit testosterone production in the testes, thus decreasing male arousal and sexual performance[77]. In women, the situation is opposite as alcohol consumption increases the production of testosterone[78]. Since testosterone controls in part the libido in women, alcohol consumption in women can increase their interest in sex. Furthermore the desinhibition factor makes women feel more relaxed which makes the whole sexual experience more fun. Since women have a higher percentage of body fats than men, alcohol will take longer to be degraded/excreted. This means that their libido can remain higher for some time as compared to men upon consumption of alcohol.

However, alcohol has many negative consequences on the body which explains why most guys prefer having most of the time sober female partners[79].

---

[77] To be more precise this will increase difficulty in attaining orgasm and will decrease overall pleasure, not to mention difficulties to get a decent boner.

[78] Yes, women also produce testosterone, although of course in much less quantities than men, In the case of women, testosterone is produced by the adrenal glands (above the kidneys) as well as the ovaries.

[79] So from a guy's perspective, the idea is basically to get a woman a little drunk to seduce her (it will also lower her standards) and once she's "hooked" to keep her sober. Genius. Of course, if you are trying to seduce the girl and want her to drink without getting yourself drunk, the ideal is to prepare some cocktails in the kitchen (e.g. whiskey coca-cola) and to

The intoxication properties of alcohol over time are very dangerous as alcohol will change the metabolism of the brain and liver[80]. Alcohol is a carcinogen and can cause several types of cancer, not limited to liver cancer, but also including mouth, pharyngeal, bowel or breast cancer. As you know, these are among the very fatal types of cancers.

Over time, brain damage from alcohol can include, memory loss and impairment of cognitive functions (ability to think) and can increase risk of other neurological diseases. It has to be noted that since women will need more time to eliminate alcohol from their bodies, they are more likely than men to get the medical problems associated with alcohol.

Alcohol also increases insulin production which can cause low sugar levels in the blood. Alcohol also has the "unexpected" property of dehydrating the body as it limits the production of a hormone called "vasopressin" which leads to a high concentration of water in urine and in vomit (when this occurs).

From a nutrition point of view, since alcohol is a highly energetic molecule, when the body will ingest it, the body will focus on generating energy in priority through the alcohol molecules. Therefore the body will not use the other carbohydrates, thus stocking them as fat. This is why regular alcohol makes people fat. In addition alcohol decreases the absorption of certain nutrients (including proteins) by the intestines. This is why regular alcohol consumption leads to nutritional deficiencies.

For men, there is an interesting long term consequence of alcohol consumption: "bitch tits" also known as "man boobs (moobs)" or medically speaking "gynecomastia" whose definition is the enlargement of breast tissues in males. Indeed, all men produce

---

pour in her glass a lot of whiskey while you put none in yours. Double genius. Disclaimer: make sure she's consenting. Otherwise you may finish in prison where you may end up becoming your cell mate's "girlfriend" which is, in most cases, not the primary objective.
[80] Liver cirrhosis is a disease often due to alcohol abuse. In this disease, liver tissue is replaced by scar tissue which cannot perform the regular activities of the liver. Liver failure is a cause of death.

estrogens, in the same way women also produce testosterone. In men, estrogens are produced by the adrenal glands. Estrogens do not only have reproductive functions but are also used for liver functions, brain functions, bone density, blood flow, etc.

Since in men alcohol decreases testosterone levels and that the estrogen production remains constant, regular alcohol drinkers will develop gynecomastia which just looks awful. Unlike women breasts, moobs tend to be saggy. The increase sensitivity of the nipples is definitely not worth it and probably most women or gay guys are not attracted by a man playing with his tits. While heavy cases of gynecomastia can be successfully operated, most milder cases of gynecomastia can be reversed by stopping alcohol consumption, reducing saturated fat consumption and very regular exercising at the gym.

Among the saddest and most dangerous consequence of alcohol consumption is fetal alcohol syndrome which is one of the consequences that can affect the fetus of a woman drinking alcohol. Fetal alcohol syndrome (FAS) is a long list of conditions that the fetus can develop due to alcohol and that are irreversible/permanent. This is due to the fact that the fetus's liver isn't fully functional before three months, which means that at the beginning of the pregnancy alcohol cannot be eliminated quickly enough from the fetus's blood. Therefore alcohol will affect the development of the brain and the organs in a irreversible manner.

FAS can lead to the baby's physical and mental development. Babies (and children or adults) with FAS often have facial deformities which are quite evident: small head, smooth area between the nose and the lips, thinner upper lip, etc. FAS also can include other physical conditions such as hearing problems, teeth and mouth malformations, liver damage, kidney and heart defects, muscular problems, hormonal disorders. The mental conditions include learning difficulties, problems with language, lack of appropriate socialization skills, poor concentration and coordination, etc.

The basic rule is no alcohol during pregnancy. If you are pregnant, do absolutely consult your medical doctor on this topic. Same advice if you are trying to get pregnant. If you think you may be pregnant go consult your medical doctor and do a pregnancy test[81].

15.4. In-depth look at postulate #2: "Focus on the difference in between calorie intake and calories spent"

A problem with many diets it that they get people focused on how much calories they take. However what really matters is the difference between the calories eaten and the calories spent that really matters.

Therefore the Smart Diet™ says that you can eat everything (postulate 1) and in whatever quantity you want (postulate 2) as long as there is a balance that makes sense in between the calories that you eat and those that you spend. If you do a lot of physical exercise you can eat much more (and be in better shape) than a couch potato feeding on rice and vegetables.

It's quite obvious that only focusing on the nutrition/diet part of the equation without looking at the physical part side of things will only lead to failure.

Indeed, physical exercise is necessary to help strengthen the body. I already talked in part 2 of this book about the benefits of exercise for the cardio-vascular system, lungs, bones, articulations, muscles, tendons, etc. Regular physical exercise[82] also helps improve the

---

[81] Early symptoms of pregnancy can include missed period, headaches, tender breast (due to hormonal changes), nausea, frequent urination, lower backaches, darkening areolas, food cravings/food aversions. Note that some women will have light bleeding very early in the pregnancy, around the time the period is due, and that can be mistaken for a period. This is called the "implantation bleeding" which is caused by the fertilized egg going into the blood-rich uterus. This usually just lasts one day or two.

[82] Only "excessive" physical exercise can weaken the immune system. Excessive physical exercise is quite rare and would be like going to the fitness twice a day, 6 times per week. Excessive physical exercise occurs only when the body doesn't have the time to recoup after a exercise. For most people, excessive physical exercise is not really something that

immune system by stimulating the production of antibodies and hormones and helps reduce the level of oxidative stress in the body.

In addition regular physical exercise will also help evacuate some of the "poor quality" nutrients we absorb. Since we will inevitably end up eating simple sugars, saturated fats or transfats, etc, it's vital that we are still to able to eliminate them from the body. This is why regular physical exercise is vital.

Physical exercise is therefore a means to remedy to our imperfect diets and lifestyles by evacuating dangerous substances from the body.

Physical exercise is therefore the "safeguard" built-in to eliminate some of the dangerous stuff we end up eating. Without physical exercise, the accumulation over time of dangerous substances (saturated fats, salt, etc.) as well as a frequent state of high oxidative stress will end up provoking the medical problems mentioned in this book which range from cancer to cerebral/vascular accidents, from erectile dysfunction to Alzheimer, from high blood pressure to Parkinson's' disease, etc.

When looking at physical exercise, there are basically two types of physical exercises.

1. Endurance training, also called "cardio",
2. Strength training, referred to as "bodybuilding".

Do bear in mind that each person is different and will react differently to what they eat and what they do (exercise). You will need to find out what works best for you. As far as morphology, we can distinguish three types of bodies:

---

they will encounter. Most people who get tired after some kind of sport are usually just out of shape.

- The ectomorphs: these people are usually skinny and have difficulties gaining weight (including muscle). In sports, they tend to rank high on endurance, flexibility and agility.

- The mesomorphs: these are the "normal" people, neither skinny nor fat. In sports, they tend to rank high on strength, speed, power and endurance.

- The endomorphs: these are the people who tend to put weight quickly (both muscle and fat) and that tend to have higher levels of body fat.

Of course, it's the last two groups which will have to focus the most on weight loss, while the first one will have greater difficulties building up muscles. You will have to determine which group you belong too as it will influence how much cardio you will need to do (see below).

15.4.1. A few words on cardio training

As said in chapter 3.1., when the body needs energy, it will use the energy sources available in the following order:

1) First, use the sugar which circulates in the blood stream.

2) If this is not enough, use the glycogen from the liver and the muscle cells and generate energy.

3) If this is not enough, use the lipids (fats) and transform them into energy.

4) If this is not enough, use the proteins from muscles to transform them into energy

The first step can last roughly 30 seconds. This is why we can for run without breathing for a few seconds: the sugar in the blood stream is sufficient to cover our energy needs. The second step can last 10 to 15 minutes depending on each individual and the intensity of the physical effort. Endurance training starts here, and corresponds to the third step which is the one that converts (burns) the fats (lipids) into energy.

Regular "cardio type" exercises will force the body to adapt to the increase level of activity and will have the following positive impacts.

1. Cardio will slightly increase pulmonary capacity

While lung capacity is hereditary, it can be slightly improved. Through cardio, the strength and endurance of the lung tissue and surrounding muscles increases. Thus a greater volume of air can be inhaled and exhaled.

When looking at pulmonary capacity one talks about VO2 max which is the maximum amount of oxygen that you can take in. It is measured by the amount of milliliters of oxygen per kilo of body weight that can you can inhale over a period of one minute. Healthy young men and women generally have a VO2 Max of 45 to 55 while trained athletes can get to 70 or higher. Regular cardio can increase your VO2 max by 5-15% which means that a single breath of air will help you get more oxygen. Needless to say that if you smoke, your VO2 max will be greatly diminished over time.

2. Cardio will increase the efficiency of oxygen absorption into the blood

This is also an important point. While the lung size cannot change, its efficiency can be improved through cardio. Indeed, training increases the number of capillaries in the lungs, allowing more oxygen to be absorbed with each breath taken. So if you do regular cardio, when you breathe, not only will you inhale more oxygen, but a greater part of the oxygen that has gone in the lungs will end up in the blood.

3. Cardio will decrease the pulse of the heart and blood pressure

This is a consequence of points 1 and 2 above. If there is more oxygen that goes in the blood, there is less need for the heart to pump quickly. This is turn will reduce blood pressure, and as you know, high blood pressure can be a cause for heart problems. Take the example of water going through a pipe. If the water has a low debit, it is not really going to affect the borders of the pipe in which it flows. However, if the pressure is great, the water could actually start damaging the interior of the pipe through erosion. In the human body, erosion of blood vessels can lead to small hemorrhages with blood clots (thrombosis) then circulating in the blood stream. If there is sufficient atherosclerosis with clogged arteries, this can lead to a heart attack or a cerebral vascular accident.

Cycling and swimming are the best cardio exercises in my opinion. Indoor cycling at the gym is safe as you are not on the road and you can focus only on your effort without fearing for cars or other stuff on the streets. Swimming is of course the king of cardio sports as it also strengthens the body. However not everybody has a swimming pool near by.

A lot of people like to jog and run outside. I understand them. It's fun, really helps you air your ideas and is cheap. The problem with running is that on the long run, all the mini shocks that occur each time a foot reaches the ground will end up damaging little by little some of the cartilage tissues in the body, in particular the spinal discs and knee cartilage. This is why many long-time runners, even those with good shoes and running on grass/soft land, end up with knee pains and/or lower back pains.

As said previously, cartilage cannot be healed. Sure you can have your knees or spinal discs replaced, but you will never recover the shape you had before. This is why I do not recommend frequent running or jogging for cardio. Sorry for all you joggers. Remember, the idea behind this book is that being healthy is a marathon, not a sprint. You don't want to be healthy until 50 years old and then you have to stop sports as your damaged knees and/or back no longer allow you to do any kind of physical exercise[83].

Okay so I may get a lot of "hate mail" from the chorus of running fanatics or from the sport apparel companies that sell overpriced shoes to a bunch of cuckoos. That doesn't bother me. Come back when in ten years and challenge me for a sprint. I'm pretty sure I will get the last laugh.

15.4.2. A few words about strength training and bodybuilding

Okay, a lot of you guys and girls may have a lot of preconceived ideas against bodybuilding or bodybuilders. Many people find the amount of muscle of the pro bodybuilders as unattractive[84]. Often I hear men and women saying that they do not want to do bodybuilding as they are "afraid to become as big" as the pros. Of course, this is nonsense. Sure, the pros do a lot of bodybuilding, but they also take a lot of drugs (steroids, human growth hormones, testosterone, insulin, diuretics, etc.) to get as big as they are. Even if you went to the gym every day of the week, there is no chance of ending as big as a pro.

However, with a lot of dedication, healthy eating and hard work, you could end up with a physique resembling those of the ancient Greek or Roman statues (male or female), which are quite esthetic according to most people. Sure, some people will always downplay your efforts. But remember that humans are envious by nature. Therefore many people will tend to belittle or "downgrade" a person with a good physique by trying to find silly arguments such as:

- "I'm sure he/she takes steroids to be like that".

---

[83] As goes the saying "once your back goes, you never come back".
[84] Less so in parts of the gay community where good looks can be very important and muscular guys are considered "hot".

- "He/she must be unemployed to have so much time to spend at the gym".

- "I could have that kind of body if I didn't have a job and a family".

All this is rubbish of course. The reality is that people are always jealous of people that they perceive as more successful than them. As the cowards say "if you cannot be better than them, criticize them when their back is turned".

The bottom line here is that if you are organized in your training and do it properly on a regular basis, results will show:

- Your muscles will grow in size and strength, therefore removing back pains and other pains.

- Your ligaments, tendons will strengthen, your cartilages will get more blood flow thus improving their condition.

- Your immune system will be better and you will be sick less often.

- Your skin will be firmer (no sagging arms or booties for women).

- Your self-confidence will be higher.

- Your cardiovascular system will be better (including better erections for the guys[85]).

- Your physique will be more pleasing to look and you will have more success with other guys or woman or both depending into what you are.

---

[85] Yeah, it's a cheap argument. But probably the one that will resonate the best in most guys' heads.

There are many books about fitness and bodybuilding, and this book is not one of them. You also can find countless videos on internet where people will explain what exercises to do and how to do them.

In a nutshell, here are some of the rules:

1. Try to go the gym at least three times per week:

    -   One day for back and biceps,
    -   One day for pecs, triceps and shoulders,
    -   One day for legs and abs.

2. If you can go to the gym more than tree times per week, you can increasingly focus your workouts on a particular muscle group.

3. Ensure each muscle group has at least 3 days of rest before the next workout (one full week is better).

4. Ensure you get enough rest (i.e. sleep at least 7-9 hours per night).

5. Drink a lot of water (at least 1 liter of water per workout)[86].

6. Proper nutrition is key so that you body can recoup and grow from the workouts.

Doing cardiovascular exercise is great. But it's quite useless to have a good heart condition if you cannot do anymore sport because your muscles are weak, your articulations damaged with arthritis or if you have chronic back pains.

This is why cardio and bodybuilding are complementary. Doing only one and not the other will only ensure problems in the future. If you don't know how to exercise at the gym, you can find many useful resources on the internet. You can also check out with a coach at

---

[86] Strong headaches can be due to the dehydration or lack of hydration following an intense physical workout session.

your local gym. There are many variants in strength training. Some focus more on weight loss through high intensity workouts, others will focus on stamina or strengthening of the core muscles (those of the abdominal belt: abdominals, obliques, lombard muscles).

If you do other sports or physical exercises, of course keep doing them, but remember their potential dangers. I am not going to go through all sports, just some of the most common.

- Tennis: over time usually ends by damaging knees (cartilage and ligaments) and elbows (cartilage).

- Jogging: over time usually ends up damaging knees (cartilage and ligaments), as well as the back (spinal discs).

- Soccer: over time over time usually ends up damaging knees (cartilage and ligaments).

- Skiing: over time usually ends up damaging knees (cartilage and ligaments).

As said, I am not recommending you to stop doing these sports if you're doing them. The message is that you need to bear in mind the risk factors and try to manage them. This includes strengthening certain body parts when certain articulations are put under severe contribution. In other cases such as jogging, you may need to reduce the frequency of doing this activity. In the case of soccer or ski the risks of significant damage to the articulations is high (whether by accident or by wearing off the articulation). This has to be also taken into consideration.

Of course, warm-up is key before doing any kind of sport to help avoid injuries. For the same reason, stretching at the end of a physical exercise is useful. In addition, bodybuilding and the strengthening of the muscles, ligaments and tendons of the areas used in the sport activity that you do are key to help avoid injuries.

Time to end this section on physical exercise, but remember the following saying:

"Today I will do what you choose not to do,
so tomorrow I can do what you no longer can do",
unknown elite sportsman

15.5. In-depth look at postulate #3: "it's a lifestyle, not a diet"

Diets are usually followed for short periods. But who wants to be in shape for only a short period of time? The Smart Diet™ is not a diet. It is a lifestyle, a way of life that you can follow all along your life.

This is why it has safeguards built within the system, i.e. the Smart Diet™ takes into account that we are human and not perfect at all times. We all know that we will deviate from the "ideal" direction. Not only does the Smart Diet™ take this into consideration, it also shows how to get back on track. It's because it already includes some degree of failure and that it proposes corrective measures that the Smart Diet™ is not a diet but really a way of life.

In next chapter, you will see how the Smart Diet™ actually works.

Chapter 16: How to implement the Smart Diet™?

This chapter explains from a practical way the how the Smart Diet™ is structured and implemented, as well as some of the "best practices". You will see, it's easy.

16.1. Determining your health/weight objectives

The first thing is to determine what your health/weight loss objectives are. Obviously depending on your objectives the implementation of the Smart Diet™ will differ from person to person. To simplify things we can distinguish between three types of objectives which I call "red zone", "yellow zone" and "green zone".

From a practical point of view, there are no differences in the implementations of these diets except for the amount of physical exercise necessary. Yups you read well, no differences in the eating habits.

Red zone:

If you want to lose a lot of fat and/or gain muscle (over 15% of your initial starting weight), you are in the "red zone". Your objective is highly ambitious and will require you to do the following:

1. Consume only "healthy" foods and drinks as those mentioned in chapter 15.3.1 with the exception of your cheat meals.

2. You are allowed a maximum of 2 cheat meals and 2 cheat "snacks/breakfasts" per week (see 16.2. below).

3. Physical exercises: at least 5 sessions per week, including at least 2 sessions of cardio (minimum 45 minutes). Even if you are seeking to lose weight, you need to do at least 3 sessions of bodybuilding in order to strengthen muscles, firm up your skin and flesh, and improve the health of your articulations.

Yellow zone:

If you want to lose some fat and/or gain muscle (5-10% of your initial starting weight), you are in the "yellow zone". Your objective is ambitious and will require you to do the following:

1. Consume only "healthy" foods and drinks as those mentioned in chapter 15.3.1 with the exception of your cheat meals.

2. You are allowed a maximum of 2 cheat meals and 2 cheat "snacks/breakfasts" per week (see 16.2. below).

3. Physical exercises: at least 4 sessions per week, including at least 2 sessions of cardio (minimum 45 minutes). Even if you are seeking to lose a more limited amount of weight, you need to do at least 2 sessions of bodybuilding in order to strengthen muscles, firm up your skin and flesh, and improve the health of your articulations.

Green zone:

In this case you have reached the "adequate" weight for your size and age.

By adequate, I mean the weight that you would like to achieve. But be ambitious! Don't aim for the "normal weight" that you should have according to your doctor based on a sample of today's "mediocre" world. Aim to have a physique and weight that is better than 80% of your peer group.

Take my case, I don't want to have a "normal" weight according to guys of my age group. I want to look better than 80% of the guys who are ten years younger than me. I want to look healthy, big, strong and ripped. I am not going to accept having a belly or a flat chest because it's "normal" in our sedentary society. I want to make Daniel Craig look like a skinny wimp. I want to make Ryan Gosling look like a bag of potatoes if he were walking next to me. You get the point.

If you're a girl, you want to look better than 80% of the other girls of your age. You want to have firm legs and arms with a strong back and a nice firm booty. And don't bring up the excuse that you have had children. The weight gained in pregnancy is not permanent.

In the green zone, you are either happy with your current weight or seek to lose less than 5% of your initial starting weight. Your objective here is more "maintenance" and it will require you to do the following:

1. Consume only "healthy" foods and drinks as those mentioned in chapter 15.3.1 with the exception of your cheat meals.

2. You are allowed a maximum of 2 cheat meals and 2 cheat "snacks/breakfasts" per week (see 16.2. below).

3. Physical exercises: at least 3 sessions per week, including at least 1 session of cardio (minimum 45 minutes). The two bodybuilding sessions are necessary to maintain the health of the muscles, tendons, bones and articulations.

16.2. Organizing meals and "cheat meals"

As said in chapter 15.2, cheat meals are an important feature in the Smart Diet™. Indeed, all long term planning must include some degree of "failure" and a road map plans to recover from these mistakes. For example, if you have a car with a GPS system and make a mistake on your way, no problem. The system will automatically readjust and set a new route for you to make sure that you reach your objective. Many diets are just tyrannical systems which, as we saw in chapter 12, are often unhealthy and sometimes outright dangerous.

As mentioned in chapter 12.2.2. one of the big problems of diets is that they are "all or nothing". They impose some crazy stuff on those who follow them. And the end is always the same: cravings increase until the moment that you are no longer able to resist the temptation and finish in front of your fridge at 01:30 AM eating everything you can put your hands on. The problem is not even the fact that you eat, the problem is that this will create a sense of guilt and shame and the idea that you are worthless, incapable of resisting temptation and unable to reach your own goals. This psychological spiral of shame and loss of self esteem will only lead you to eat more than before and even less capable of improving your lifestyle and nutrition habits.

This is why "cheat meals" are such an import part of the Smart Diet™. Cheat meals have the following benefits:

1. They avoid accumulating frustrations or cravings that end up with binge eating and the ensuing spiral of loss of self esteem.

2. They motivate you to eat and drink "healthy" the rest of the time (i.e. 80% of the time).

3. They ensure that the Smart Diet™ becomes your lifestyle rather than a diet.

4. They become a "pleasurable treat" which you can really look forward to and enjoy without any sense of shame. They are your reward you for eating healthy 80% of the time and for doing regular physical exercise.

So how do you organize cheat meals?

Chapter 15.3.2 includes a list of "poor quality" foods and drinks while chapter 15.3.3 includes a list of foods which are harmful if eaten in great quantities or at high frequencies.

The idea is that you take eat two cheat meals per week as well as two cheat breakfasts or snacks per week. This makes up for two "big" cheat meals and two "smaller" cheat meals. You choose when you want to take the cheat meals. You can take them the same day or split them more evenly in the week. In order to not build up any cravings it's actually a good idea not to set fixed days for your cheat meals but to take them when you want. So if it's the week-end and you feel like having a BBQ with beer, go ahead. If in the morning you want to have eggs and bacon together with a burger and fries, go ahead. What counts is that at the end of the week, out of the 21 meals you had, there are at least 17 which were "quality" meals with "quality" foods and "quality" drinks. Therefore, when you do a cheat meal, the important thing is that you are not left with a craving. Of course, you don't want to eat until the point you get sick and vomit, but you should not end a cheat meal with a craving or a sense of frustration[87].

As mentioned previously, you can choose to try to offset a cheat meal by consuming foods or drinks with high antioxidant levels. For example, especially in Europe, you could choose to have a glass or two of red wine with red meat or a BBQ. You could also choose to have an apple after eating a pack of chocolate cookies or brownies[88].

Also, you are not obliged to eat all the cheat meals of the week. In summer, people often like to eat lighter, and you may choose not to have the two cheat meals you are entitled too. However, if one week you only take one "big" cheat meal, you cannot decide that the next week you are entitled to three big cheat meals. In no case can you take more than the two big and the two small cheat meals.

So you see, cheat meals are essential for the Smart Diet™. They are easy to manage as you choose how to go about them. The only rule

---

[87] Within reason, of course.
[88] If you're lucky enough to know someone knows how to cook good brownies.

is no more than two "big" and two "smaller" cheat meals per week. And to set the record straight, snacking is considered as a "small" cheat meal.

16.3. Organizing your sessions of physical exercise

Here also, there are no rules but just common sense. You choose when you want to do your cardio or your bodybuilding sessions. You can do them first thing in the morning, over lunch or after work depending on what suits you best.

Common sense suggests that you try to include a day of rest in between your workout/cardio days. In the case that you are in the "red zone" and doing at least 5 sessions of sport per week you can of course not allow a day of rest in between each session. It's up to you to see how you want to manage your resting days. Personally, for my bodybuilding sessions, I choose to do a different muscle group each session. For example, on Monday I will do pecs, Tuesdays biceps, Wednesday legs, Fridays back and Saturday shoulders. This allows me do have a full week of rest for each muscle group. So even if Tuesday my pecs are sore from Monday's workout, it doesn't matter as I will not solicit them until the following Monday.

Rest is essential for muscles and articulations. In fact if you want to build muscle strength and strengthen articulations and tendons, you need to do the following three things:

1. Eat well,
2. Drink well,
3. Rest well (including sleep).

Not doing one or the other of these three points will not enable the body to recoup, regenerate and rebuild itself. This is how injuries occur. So remember, exercise, eat, drink and rest. That's the way to stay injury free. Each body is different, so listen to your body and determine what works the best for you, especially as far as the resting part. This is a nice transition for the next section.

16.3. Sleep

Sleep is important and not only on weekends. In fact sleep is essential. Everybody knows that a lack of eating or drinking are fatal. Few people realize that a lack of sleep also leads to death. But before you sleep right away, please read the following section ☺.

Sleep is a state characterized by a reduced consciousness as well as a decreased reactivity to external stimuli. During sleep there is an inactivity of nearly all voluntary muscles. This is provoked by the production of certain hormones that will inhibit the neurons related to motor activities, i.e. movements other than those that are necessary and that continue at night (heart beats, diaphragm, etc).

Sleep paralysis is a condition that can be recurring (or not) whereby some people wake up and are conscious but are unable to move. This is the case when sleep cycles are perturbed and the mind wakes up while the production of motor inhibiting hormones has not ended. This condition can last a few seconds or a few minutes and can be scary for those experiencing it for the first time[89]. Of course any case of sleep paralysis requires to consult with a medical doctor.

16.3.1. Sleep hours and the circadian clock

The timing of sleep is regulated by the "circadian clock" and other mechanisms which regulate the sleep-awake cycle. What is amazing it that the area of the brain (bottom central area) which is responsible for managing our biological clock is comprised "only" of approximately 20'000 neurons out of the over 80 billion[90] that a brain is said to have. In this area of the brain (called suprachiasmatic nuclei), the neurons use among others stimuli from other senses (especially light) to determine what time it is.

---

[89] Generally only the eyes can be controlled in a phase of sleep paralysis. A person in this state will however not be able to talk.

[90] 80 billion is a lot. This means that the brain has almost as many neurons as the Milky Way galaxy has of stars.

It's this clock that makes that you feel tired about at the same time everyday, go to the bathroom at about the same time every day, etc. This clock also determines hormone production, body temperature, cell division, etc. Our biological clock regulates all the processes which are function of time. The circadian clock is said to be so precise that it only deviates by a maximum of a few minutes per day. The biological clock of humans is said to be 24 hours and 11 minutes +/- 16 minutes on average.

The following image from Wikipedia shows how the body's functions can change depending on the time of the day.

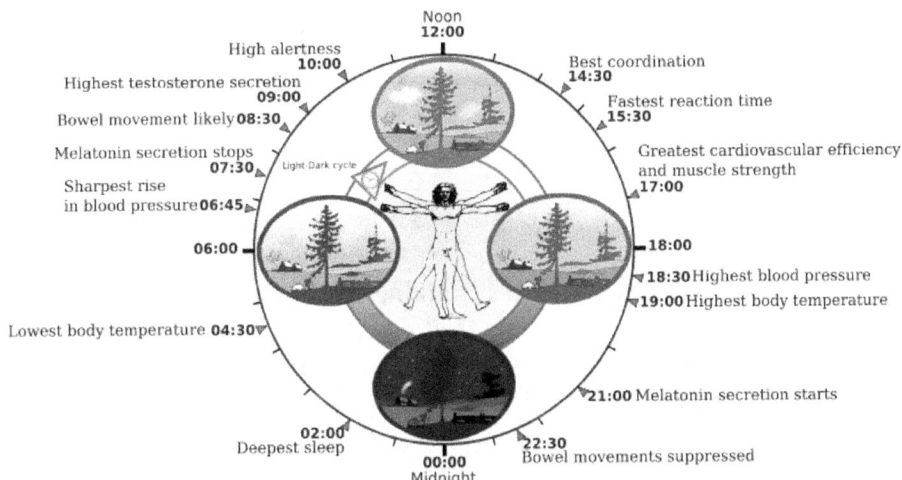

Source: Wikipedia

Some of these facts are well known. For example we all know fever is highest the evenings and guys probably know they get stiff in the mornings. We also know the "quality" sleep occurs after midnight and not a 5:00 AM coming back from the club.

As we all know, sleeping requirements change with age.

Age and condition	Sleep Needs
Newborns (0–2 months)	12 to 18 hours
Infants (3–11 months)	14 to 15 hours
Toddlers (1–3 years)	12 to 14 hours
Preschoolers (3–5 years)	11 to 13 hours
School-age children (5–10 years)	10 to 11 hours
Adolescents (10–17 years)	8.5 to 9.25 hours
Adults, including elderly	7 to 9 hours

Source: Wikipedia

As said previously, sleep is a highly "anabolic[91]" state where the body will repair itself and grow. But there are many functions of sleep:

16.3.2. The different functions of sleep

1. Restoration, healing and repairing the body

The state of sleep is highly anabolic, which means that it's a state where the nutrients absorbed by the body are more efficiently used to restore/repair the body.

The human growth hormone (HGH) is one that enables growth in children to get to their adult sizes. We know that the growth process requires a lot of sleep as the anabolic state is the one that increases the speed of restoration, repair and growth. Few people do realize that HGH is produced throughout life, i.e. even in adults. Indeed, every day the body has to repair damage sustained during the day by the oxidation of molecules, as well as by the many small damages/lesions incurred.

---

[91] Anabolic means that the body in a state of (re)building current structures with the nutrients absorbed. Catabolic is the opposite, whereby certain structures progressively lose some of their mass/density due to a lack of nutrients.

What is interesting is that 50% of daily HGH production occurs one hour after falling asleep and essentially in between midnight and 4:00 AM. This explains why sleeping very late (e.g. after a night of clubbing) leads to a state of fatigue independently of the hours slept. Indeed, if the production on HGH over the period of sleep is lower, the body will have had less time to repair itself. In addition, studies have shown that deprived sleep negatively affects the immune system through lower counts of white cells and other elements of the immune system. This explains why sleep is important to heal from wounds or illnesses. This is why people who are ill or wounded tend to feel tired and sleep more. It also explains why people who are tired are at more risk to catch colds and other illnesses[92].

From a nutrition point of view, it is also interesting to know that as long as the body produces insulin, it will not produce HGH. These hormones cannot be produced at the same time.

Why is this important? Well say that you go to a night club and have a sandwich before returning home, or if you just choose to have a late fancy meal at 23:00 before going to bed, the body will produce insulin to absorb the sugars which get into the blood. As this part of the digestion can last 1-2 hours, it means that during 1 or 2 hours no HGH will be produced. Therefore going to bed right away after eating means that you will not produce HGH at the beginning of your sleep. So although you could be in your deep sleep period, no HGH will be produced and the body will not be able to repair itself well, thus leading to fatigue the next day and greater chances of getting ill or sustaining injuries of muscles, articulations, etc.

HGH production at adults is a little more than 60% of those of young adolescents. Natural stimulators of HGH include deep sleep, vitamin B3, as well as physical exercise.

---

[92] I am not saying not to go clubbing or to the restaurant, but just to ensure you get adequate rest over a week.

2. Memory processing

Studies show that sleep improves the process whereby information is memorized.

3. Brain development (for infants)

It has been shown that sleep is necessary for the development of the brain of infants. Indeed, during sleep the brain is able to develop by activating synapses (neuron transmitters) without any motor (movement) consequences for the child. Sleep deprivation for infants can lead to a decreased brain mass, behavior problems and abnormal neural cell death.

The lack of sleep is therefore a dangerous condition for infants and adults. The chart bellows indicates some of the effects of sleep deprivation.

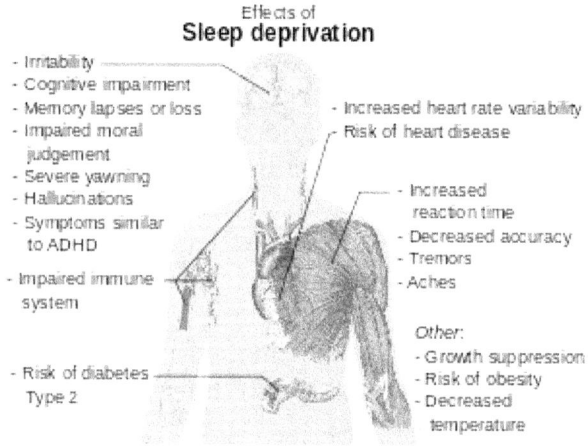

Source: Wikipedia

16.3.3. Other issues on the subject of sleep

1. Sleep disorders

Insomnia (difficulties to fall asleep) or narcolepsy (brain's inability to regulate sleep-awake state) are serious conditions which need medical help.

Snoring is a cause of sleep deprivation and can lead to irritability, lack of focus or decreased libido. There is also a link between loud snoring and heart attack as the tongue can block airway passage into the lungs and therefore create a state of apnea. Sleep apnea can be a dangerous and sometimes fatal condition. Obesity can be a cause of sleep apnea. In other cases, sleep apnea can be due to the structure of the jaw bone relative to the skull. Surgery is sometimes required for life threatening cases. In lighter cases, people may need to use a facial mask and or a machine to help them breathe during their sleep (continuous positive airway pressure machine).

2. Substances that can disturb sleep

Some substances can induce sleepiness and are in some cases used to help against insomnia. However some of them can have negative secondary effects:

- Alcohol: impacts sleep cycles and leads over time to insomnia,

- Marijuana: impacts deep sleep (and therefore HGH production among others).

Other substances are known as stimulants and reduce sleepiness. They often lead to issues of insomnia and/or sleep cycle disorders.

- Caffeine: no need to say more on this one.

- Cocaine/amphetamines: can lead to significant disorders in the circadian cycle.

- Tobacco: disrupts sleep cycles and has been found to reduce total sleep time.

3. Other factors which can affect sleep disorders

Shift work (i.e. working at night), jet lags or even pregnancy can affect the circadian rhythm. Certain drugs or medicines also affect the biological clock. Aging is another factor.

16.3.4. Closing remarks on sleep

As discussed above, sleep is a complex process that involves slight changes in body temperature and hormone production in order to favor anabolism. Any long lasting trend of lack of sleep (sleep deprivation) or any lasting trend of sleep cycle disorders will inevitably lead to an accelerated aging process as the body is not able to repair itself sufficiently. It will also induce a weaker immune system.

Every person has different sleep requirements, and the idea is certainly not to sleep as much as possible[93]. However the idea is to sleep well, i.e. that the body is given enough time to repair itself. As seen above certain substances can disturb a quality sleep. A partner's snoring can be another factor that disturbs quality sleep, which is why loud snoring can become a health issue for both partners.

---

[93] To the opposite, too much sleep is dangerous as it has been linked to increased risks of heart diseases, obesity and diabetes.

Quality sleep cycles require a certain stability in patterns. This is why it is preferable to have a certain routine before going to sleep, such as going to bed more or less at the same time every week day or taking 15-30 minutes before going to bed to relax and decrease your level of activity. Since luminosity is one of the key stimulus' used by the body to determine the time, it's recommended to shut off computers, televisions, tablets, phones and other electronic devices at least 15 minutes before going to bed. Simply reading a few minutes can help decrease the level of activity of the body to better prepare it to fall asleep as quickly as possible.

Sleep disorders can be serious medical conditions. Do not take any medicine to help you sleep without having consulted a medical doctor first.

I will not get into further details of the sleep cycles as it gets out of the scope of this book. If you are interested in this subject you will find many resources available, but some of the main topics of sleep have been addressed in this chapter.

I will not get either into the subject of dreams as it's also out of the scope of this book. I will however end this section with a fun fact on dreams. In their dreams, men dream more about men than women will dream about women. Why? I have no clue! Go figure it out! If one of you readers is a psychologist, please let me know why.

16.4. Follow-up

The Smart Diet™ is just about common sense. It's important that you try to follow your routine as far as eating and doing physical exercise. Monitor your weight daily. Look at your self in the mirror naked and check your progress. Progress always follows a similar pattern which resembles a staircase:

- There is a first period which is tough and during which the body has not adapted to the new lifestyle. You will not see gains in this period which can last 4-8 weeks.

- Once the body realizes that the changes in nutrition and physical habits are not a "one off", non-recurring event, but a permanent change in lifestyle, gains show up fast. You gain strength, build muscle and start losing fat. You have walked one step up the staircase.

- There is a "plateau" or period of stabilization where the body consolidates its weight to the new "state" of the health. Weight losses and muscle gains slow.

- Through your continuous physical exercise and proper nutrition, your muscles gain further strength and you burn more fats. Weight losses and muscle gains accelerate again as you walk another step up the staircase.

The process of alternating a period of stabilization and then a period of muscle gain/weight loss then continues until you reach the "green zone" where you have reached your weight targets (fat and muscle) and where you get into a mode of maintenance and stabilization.

Do note that the body doesn't like big changes in weight in particular if the direction fluctuates both ways. I.e. having periods of weight gains and losses is really bad for the heart and the internal organs who get "confused" and have a hard time to adapt to an ever changing situation that will require different levels of activity.

This is why it's important to implement and keep the Smart Diet™ in order to ensure that fat loss and muscle gains go in one direction. As this happens, the different organs will be less solicited and will be able to rest more and be in better health. Remember that if an organ has to do "too much" effort for "too long", it will eventually shut down.

For example, a poor nutrition and lifestyle will oblige (among others):

- The heart to pump more often which can lead to hypertension (significant risk factor for cardiovascular diseases).

- The liver to be much more involved in detoxification activities that eventually can lead to part of the liver's cells to no longer function (can lead to fatal liver failure and kidney problems).

- The pancreas cells to produce too much insulin too often (can lead to type II diabetes).

Also remember that excess activity by an organ can increase the state of oxidative stress leading to cancer. To the contrary, a heart beating slower, a liver doing less efforts for "massive" desintoxication, a pancreas secreting less insulin frequently are all beneficial conditions which will enable the organs to work properly for a much longer period of time.

Sounds simple, huh? Well it is! There is no voodoo here. Nutrition (70%) and physical exercise (30%) are the simple keys to lose fat and get in better shape. Does it take some determination? Yes. Does it entail efforts? Of course. If you think that you can get in shape with no effort or by just putting some kind of machine on your belly for 10 minutes in front of the TV, you are definitely in wonderland. And forget the ads you see on TV. All the "actors" you see are professional fitness models and I can tell you that they got their physique through proper nutrition and physical exercise (and in some cases through steroids).

So do not believe any of the dieting crap you see in the media or internet. Do not believe any diet secrets from some kind of guru or Hollywood star. Set your self free from all the hoaxes and hype flying around. Focus on nutrition and physical exercise. That's the one and only way to lose fat, get in better shape and live in better health longer. It's all about common sense which, unfortunately, is not so common anymore.

Chapter 17: Example of a Smart Diet™

Here is an example of what could be a Smart Diet™ "best practice". This is what works for my body. You will have to adapt your nutrition to what suits your body best.

17.1. Breakfast

When you wake up, your body has basically not eaten anything for 8 or 10 hours. It's important to take a lot of complex carbs which will be converted very gradually into simple sugars that go in the blood. As said above, any intake of too much simple carbs which just make your insulin jump and you will end up feeling a "sugar fatigue" later. It is also important to get some proteins as, during your sleep, the body used the proteins available to repair the damages incurred to the muscles the previous day.

In addition I recommend to take three types (not more) of food supplements:

1. Multi-vitamin and multi-mineral pills: even if you have a good diet, these make sure you don't have any deficiencies. Cycle these pills, i.e. take them for 30 or 45 days and than take 30 or 45 days off. This helps avoid any strains on the liver and kidney.

2. Fish oil pills (cod liver oil or other): the high levels of omega 3 and other essential fatty acids are extremely healthy to prevent/stabilize certain health conditions. Taking fish oil pills is especially necessary for those who do not like to eat fish. You can take these pills every day, non stop. No need to cycle them.

3. Anti-oxididant pills: I have discussed many times over the importance of anti-oxidants. While you find some in fruits and other food products, there is no harm in taking a good dose of anti-oxidants which you can find in the form of pills (often they are a concentrate of fruits and in some cases have been fermented by bacteria to increase their absorption by the intestines). Unless you have cholesterol issues, you can cycle these pills, i.e. take them for 30 or 45 days and than take 30 or 45 days off.

Do note that "supplements" mean that they are "in supplementation of" a healthy diet. Excessive intake of vitamins, minerals and other molecules will at the best create liver and kidney fatigue, at the worst they will lead to other very negative medical conditions. So the idea here is to make sure you get all the things your body needs, but not to get into harmful excessive doses. If you're not sure if you are taking too much of a supplement, read the indicated dosage on the label. Double check with the internet. Triple check with your medical doctor. Again, it's all about common sense.

Best practice morning breakfast is:

- Healthy portion of oat meal (or any other whole grain) with milk (you can put a bit of sugar or honey),
- Yogurt,
- Orange juice (for the vitamin C),
- Green tea (for the antioxidant properties),
- Multi vitamin/multi mineral pill,
- Fish oil pill,
- Antioxidant pill.

If you are lactose intolerant, you can of course find milk for lactose intolerant persons.

Whole bread is okay too, the problem is that if you add to much jam its becomes very sugary. If you start putting peanut butter, jam and Nutella, then you are definitely doing a "cheat meal" breakfast.

Pancakes or French toast are ok, but less good than oat meals/cereals due to the lack of complex carbs.

17.2. Morning snack

In the middle of the morning, it is good to eat a little to keep your energy levels high. Especially if you are doing a lot of sport.

Best practice morning snack is:

- Banana (for the simple sugars),
- For those doing a lot of sport, bars with whole cereals are a good source of carbs and proteins,
- Small potion of oat meal for those who can have access to a fridge,
- Water (0.2 liters at least).

17.3. Lunch

Lunch is an important meal as it serves to give you energy for the next 5 to 6 hours. Here you really need high quality proteins, high quality carbs and fibers.

Best practice lunch is:

- White meat (veal, chicken, turkey or fish): for a high quality protein source,
- Whole rice (or another grains) or sweet potatoes: for the complex carbs,
- Salad and vegetables: for the dietary fibers and minerals,
- Fruits: for the sugars and antioxidants,
- Water (at least 0.5 liters),
- If possible red tea (rooibos) for the antioxidants,
- A small piece of black chocolate (or regular chocolate if you find the black chocolate to bitter): for the antioxidants and positive impact on mood. The chocolate bars with caramel and other stuff, chocolate cookies are small "cheat meal"

material. Here I am talking about the regular pure chocolate bars.

Red meat is good once per week for its iron content. To avoid the high cholesterol of red meat, try dried red meat which is red meat with a very low fat level (usually less than 5%). However dried red meat should not be taken more than once per week as it can be heavy to digest, and more importantly, it has a very high salt content.

Sweet potatoes, fries, red meat, fancy sauces all belong to the category of the "big" cheat meals, not the best practice meals.

17.4. Afternoon snack

In the afternoon one often has a dip in energy, especially those that do sport over lunch. The afternoon snack is identical to the morning one

Best practice afternoon snack is:

- Banana (for the simple sugars),
- For those doing a lot of sport, bars with whole cereals are a good source of carbs and proteins,
- Small potion of oat meal for those who can have access to a fridge,
- Water (0.2 liters at least).

17.5. Diner

Diner is the last meal of the day. As said before, enough time should elapse in between the end of the diner and the beginning of sleep to ensure insulin production returns to normal levels before HGH production is scheduled. Also, a high content of dietary fibers is advised to ensure smooth digestion and intestinal transit. Some people say that at night you should have something light(er) than lunch as for some people is eases the digestion. This is really something that differs from one person to another. If this is your case, you should just avoid some of the heaver to digest grains such as lentils or beans, as well as starch rich foods.

Best practice diner is (similar to lunch):

- White meat (veal, chicken, turkey or fish): for a high quality protein source,
- Whole rice (or another grains) or sweet potatoes: for the complex carbs,
- Salad and vegetables: for the dietary fibers and minerals,
- Fruits: for the sugars and antioxidants,
- Water (at least 0.5 liters),
- If possible red tea (rooibos) for the antioxidants,
- A small (and unique) glass of red wine: for the antioxidants.

There are many sayings out there on nutrition. One says that you should have breakfast like a king/queen, lunch like a prince/princess and diner like a beggar. If you have overall healthy meals (excluding the cheat meals), and if you do regular exercise, this saying makes no sense. To the opposite, any lifestyle that can lead to hunger/starvation will only increase the odds of "binge eating". Remember too that the diner is the last meal of the day and that if you do not eat enough, the body will not have enough nutrients to build and repair itself from the damages incurred during the day.

17.6. Smart Dieting on budget

By now you know why "junk food" is not good for your health. Unfortunately, as junk food is cheap, the population that is the most financially challenged is the one that consumes the most junk food (both in fast food restaurants and prepared food bought at the supermarkets). However it does not need to be this way. While fast food can be convenient, it is possible to eat healthy while on a tight budget.

Indeed, white meat (chicken, turkey) is among the cheapest of meats. While some fish are expensive, tuna, sardines and other types of fishes are not expensive. Vegetables can also be found at low prices, as well as fruits. Water from the tap or plain water is cheaper than the sodas. Regular whole bread is probably cheaper than a pizza. A regular chocolate is cheaper than a pack of cookies and so forth. So being on a tight budget will of course impact the consumption of the "extras". But as far as the "essentials", you can find them relatively cheap, and not more expensive than the junk food. It's really a question of getting the habit of eating differently and making do without the convenience and "easy way out" of junk foods and fast food restaurants.

For those that are on the road during the day (truckers, police, ambulance, etc.) eating healthy is not easy, especially when the weather is hot, it is not easy to keep fresh food. Yet, in some cases, maybe you can put a cold chicken and rice salad with vegetables in a plastic Tupperware with a aluminum foil around it to keep it fresh. Maybe you can also carry red tea in a thermos rather than picking a gallon of soda. I didn't say it's easy, but I'm saying it's possible.

And if you do go to an inexpensive restaurant, try to avoid the "bad stuff". In most cases, you can ask for some chicken and you can ask to be served rice rather than French fries. You can also ask for water rather than a soda. You can also ask the chicken to not come with any sauce. You can ask for a regular salad. The message is here too, you can eat in an inexpensive restaurant and still eat healthy.

Lose weight now!

Part 6: Other health and nutrition topics

This part of the book will address certain other health and nutrition topics, as indeed nutrition impacts many biological processes other than those already discussed.

Lose weight now!

Chapter 18: Woman's chapter

Just when you thought that man was an unbelievably complex machine, nature decided to make things even more complicated when it created women. Indeed women have a whole extra layer of complexity due to their reproductive system which includes highly complex hormonal processes as well as other biological mechanisms.

Unfortunately for guys, nature was not able to produce this "creation" without a series of well-known "defects" commonly observed in women including: lack of sense of orientation, craving for shopping and useless stuff, the inability to make up their mind when choosing clothing or furniture as well as habit of asking questions when they already have the answer in their mind and get angry if they don't get this answer[94].

This chapter focuses more on women. If you're a guy, you can probably skip this section although it could help you better understand women. I'm joking of course: guys will never understand women. However if you're a guy you may understand some of the biological features of women.

18.1. Nutrition and menstruation

Overall nutrition is important for woman of childbearing age. Indeed, the menstruation cycle will lead to many changes in hormonal balances.

---

[94] Nah, I'm just kidding. Feminists, please do not send me hate mail! Was I kidding?

18.1.1. Iron deficiency

Iron needs are an important issue for women of childbearing age. Indeed, most women will lose approximately 0.6 deciliters of blood during their period, therefore losing a lot or iron. For women with low iron, a condition of anemia may develop. In many cases this can be avoided by taking food with high levels of iron such as dried red meat which in addition contains very little fat and a lot of proteins.

As said in chapter 4.2., taking vitamin C (such as orange juice or a vitamin C pill) while eating the dried red meat helps the absorption of the iron by the intestine. Also, avoid to take calcium at the same time as iron as this will reduce their absorption by the body. Multi-vitamin pills are also a good thing to take on a regular basis (remember to cycle them, i.e. take them every two months).

18.1.2. Premenstrual syndrome (PMS)

PMS is a condition which affects many women. PMS is linked to changes in hormone levels as well as to an increase of serotonin[95] levels in the brain. PMS is closely tied to mood swings[96], water retention, tender breasts, headaches, fatigue, anxiety, changes in libido and food cravings. PMS often appears at ovulation and disappears 14 days in to the cycle. Here too nutrition can help. Indeed, avoiding or reducing the intake of certain foods such as caffeine, simple sugars, salt, saturated fatty acids and alcohol helps reduce certain symptoms of PMS. On the other hand, stress or depression can be aggravating factors for PMS.

Vegetables, fish, complex carbs as well as high calcium foods are said to help reduce PMS symptoms. Physical exercise as well.

18.2. Nutrition and pregnancy

---

[95] Serotonin affects mood but is also used in other body processes such as bone metabolism or cardiovascular growth.
[96] Known by men as the female "bitchiness" factor.

Pregnancy leads to changes in dietary requirements. This is out of scope of this book. Should you be pregnant, consult a medical doctor who will be able to help you plan your nutrition requirements based on the following factors:

- Age,
- General state of health,
- Diseases (if any),
- Metabolism and morphology.

Some of the features of pregnancy nutrition are well known and basically are the "quality" eating advocated in this book in chapter 15.3.1:

- Drink lots of water,
- Eat lean meats (white meats, fish),
- Eat a lot of fish oils and non-saturated fatty acids,
- Eat lots of vegetables, fruits,
- Eat high levels of dietary fibers (to avoid constipation issues),
- Avoid high intakes of saturated fats but do take some (very low fat diets during pregnancy are not healthy for the fetus or the mother.

There are of course some absolute "no-nos". Avoid these substances that can put the fetus at risk and cause permanent damage:

- Avoid alcohol: will cause fetal malformations,

- Avoid smoking: increases risk of miscarriage, premature births, increases sudden infant death disease, as well as increases chances of other health conditions for the baby,

- Avoid (strongly decrease) caffeine consumption, avoid stimulants: can increase risk of miscarriage,

- Avoid consumption of drugs: will affect fetal development,

- Do not take medicines without consulting your medical doctor.

Do remember that children or adults who were exposed as fetuses to high levels of alcohol, smoking, stimulant or drug consumption by their mother will have life long sequels or health fragilities that cannot be healed. So if you're about to be a mother, don't be selfish and be extra-careful for your baby. If you have any addictions (smoking, alcohol or drugs) do talk to your medical doctor who will help you find ways to deal with your addiction during pregnancy. There is nothing sadder than seeing images of malformed or cocaine addicted babies. ☹

18.3. Libido

Contrary to what most men can think, there are actually some women who have some kind of libido, including after child birth. Libido is related to the state of mind (stress or not) as well as the state of the body (tired or not). Physical illnesses or psychological factors do affect libido.

Nevertheless some nutrients are shown to be helpful to *increase* libido[97]:

Vitamin B6: helps balance progesterone and estrogen levels. Regular consumption of B6 helps women increase orgasm and sexual stamina. B3 is also helpful for hormone production. Vitamins B6 and B3 can be found in seafood among others, as well as chicken, fish or red meat.

Vitamin C: increases fertility and overall energy levels. So eat lots of fruits!

Zinc: low zinc levels is found to be one of the leading causes of decreased libido. Multi-vitamin and multi-mineral pills contain zinc. Regular consumption of zinc should bring libido levels back to normal. Other foods which are rich in zinc include seafood, chicken, oatmeal, milk, pecans, cashews, brown rice, etc.

---

[97] Guys, now is the time to take notes.

Vitamin E: helps improve circulation as well as reduce some of the symptoms of PMS. Vitamin E can be found in almonds, pine nuts, peanuts, green olives, olive oil, cooked spinach, etc.

Regular physical exercise is also said to improve libido by increasing the release of "feel good" hormones, as well an increased sense of self-confidence. In addition to "traditional" physical exercise, you may want to try the "Kegel exercises". For those who are not familiar, the Kegel exercises can be done by men or women and consist of contracting the pelvic muscles for a few seconds and then relaxing the muscles.

Strengthening the pelvic muscles has shown the following benefits for women:

- Reducing risk of incontinence,
- Strengthening vaginal muscles helps increase orgasm,
- Good for treating vaginal prolapse (after child birth).

Kegel exercises can be done anywhere as it's totally discreet. You can do it at home or at work. An example of a Kegel routine would be the following:

a) Contract the pelvic muscles[98] for 5-8 seconds, then relax for 5 seconds (this is one repetition),

b) Do 10-15 repetitions before taking a 2 minute break (this is called one series),

c) Do a total of 3-4 series every two or three times per week.

---

[98] The pelvic muscles are the ones you contract when for example you need to retain an envy to pee.

To the contrary, certain substances *decrease* libido:

Caffeine: indeed high caffeine intake will cause adrenal fatigue[99] which will decrease the production of cortisol which helps deal with stress. In turn this will affect desire and energy for sex.

- Tobacco: due to the vasoconstriction factors which will overtime decrease the blood flow to the clitoris.

- Saturated fats: for the same reason as above, the saturated fats will lead to plague formation which, over time, will decrease blood flow to the clitoris.

These nutritional tips should help transform most women from "Nanuk, the frigid penguin from Antarctica" into "Tracy Cummings, the hot porn star from Las Vegas"[100,101].

I will end up this section with a remark destined to the guys. Ultimately the woman's libido is related to her state of mind. If her state of mind is not good, it's probably your fault, and you should be doing something about it. In most cases, it's because you are neglecting her and not caring for her physical, psychological or emotional needs.

18.4. Fertility

Infertility can be caused by genetic factors as well as illnesses. Fortunately today medicine has improved and less fertile couples can also have children with the help of medicine.

In any case, there are some foods which can increase your fertility levels and others that can decrease them. So if you are trying to conceive, do take a look at the factors below.

---

[99] Fatigue of the adrenal glands.
[100] This is of course a fictitious name. Don't search it on internet :p
[101] If this doesn't still help maybe I could do the job. However I'm afraid your boyfriend/girlfriend may not appreciate it.

Foods to take:

Iron: pregnancy requires high iron levels. Being low on iron due to periods can reduce fertility.

Omega 3 and 6s: increase intake of fish and fish oils.

Increase vitamin intake: vitamins A, folic acid and B12. Here too, the multi-vitamin pills should be enough.

Foods to avoid:

Caffeine: high levels of caffeine decrease iron and calcium absorption and negatively impact the chances of getting pregnant.

High levels of alcohol have shown to slightly decrease fertility levels in women.

High levels of refined carbs (simple sugars) will increase surges in insulin which can cause irregular ovulation. This is especially important for women with polycystic ovary syndrome. As said previously, women with this condition should focus on a higher non saturated fat intake, as well as on complex carbs. This special diet should be made under the guidance and supervision of a medical doctor.

If you have trouble conceiving do consult with a medical doctor to assess where does the problem lie. It may be due to the woman, the man or both. Remember, nutrition can only get you up to a certain point. If the problems are more significant, only medical help will provide solutions.

18.5. Menopause

Menopause is another period with big hormonal changes for women. The changes can also be mental as this is an important evolution in their life. The reduction in production of certain hormones can increase certain health risks (e.g. osteoporosis).

Generally the period before the menopause, called perimenopause, is more dramatic than the menopause itself as the changes are more significant. Here are some of the symptoms which can occur:

- Hot flashes,
- Menstrual cycle changes (heavier, lighter, frequency can change too),
- Mood changes,
- Changes in appetite (nausea, cravings),
- Sleep disturbances,
- Memory changes (reduction of estrogen can decrease the brain function of memory),
- Urinary symptoms (changes in urination frequency, slight incontinence, increased incidence of urinary tract infections due to the changes in the bacteria in the vagina),
- Decrease in libido (can be accompanied by vaginal dryness),
- Digestive disturbances (heat burns),
- Ovarian growths (there can be benign ovarian cysts).

Of course, each woman may experience one or several of these symptoms to different degrees. In all cases, women should consult with their medical doctor when going though the perimenopause and the menopause.

In these periods, nutrition should be focusing on the following to decrease some of the symptoms mentioned above:

- Increase iron intake,
- Increase calcium intake,
- Increase zinc intake,
- Increase intake of dietary fibers,
- Limit saturated fat consumption,
- Limit salt and simple sugar consumption,
- Limit alcohol intake.

Wait. It sounds familiar, no? Yes indeed, basically what is recommended for women going through menopause is the "clean" diet which I mentioned already in section 15.3.1. It's also the same as the basics for nutrition during pregnancy and the one to increase libido.

Bottom line: the Smart Diet™, is basically an all-around nutrition which you can adopt whatever your age and whatever your condition.

Chapter 19: Man's chapter

As said above, man is the simpler version of a woman. Less sophisticated, less capable of interacting with others, man is basically the version 1.0 of the human being while women are probably version 5.0 and above. It's a bit like comparing a mobile phone from the 90's to a smart phone of today.

This is why the chapter on men will be shorter, there is simply less to say.

It's often said that the value of a man is measured by the value of his acts. The reality is that men measure themselves by the strength of their erections, that's why I'll focus mainly on erections and mens' libido which usually starts at age 10-12 and ends at death[102].

19.1. Erections

Erections are triggered by the autonomic nervous system and may result from a variety of stimuli including sexual stimulation and sexual arousal as well as changes in hormone balances during sleep. From a chemical point of view, the release of nitric oxide (a vasodilator) will lead to an accumulation of blood in the sponge-like tissues (corpus cavernosum) of the penis as the arteries in the penis will dilate. At the same time muscles will compress the veins of the corpus cavernosum to restrict the outflow of blood from the penis.

Erections are closely tied to the circulatory system. However there are also psychological factors which come into play and that I will discuss below. Hormonal issues can also impact erections. Those too will be discussed below.

---

[102] If you're a girl and want to know whether your guy watches porn on his computer, here's an easy trick: if his internet browser's history is empty he is definitely watching porn.

If you're a guy, you probably want to know how you compare to others. Indeed most guys think that it's normal to have erections lasting much longer than what is real. Forget about the male porn stars, the scenes they perform in are usually recorded over several hours so in reality the guys are actually not erect non-stop.

So here is a fact: over 70% of males reach orgasm within two minutes of non-stop intercourse[103].

Of course with extra stimulation, foreplay and so forth, the erections (whether full erections or semi-erections) can last anywhere from 5 to 15 minutes. Some men have the ability to regain an erection quite quickly after a previous ejaculation and that can prolong the overall duration of sex. However this is a case of a succession of erections and not just a single long one.

Erections which last longer than 4 hours are a painful condition known as priapism which requires medical treatment. In this case, medications will be given at first. If unsuccessful, the doctors (usually urologists) will have to puncture small holes into the penis so blood can be released, ouch!

19.2. Erectile dysfunction

Erectile dysfunctions will affect at some point in time most males. There are several known causes for erectile dysfunction (ED). One however should distinguish between several situations:

- "permanent" ED versus an "occasional" ED,
- "real" ED versus a "soft erection".

A permanent ED is a medical condition that requires consulting with a medical doctor, and in some cases, with a specialist (urologist). Since there are medical causes which are responsible for the ED, medical help is needed.

---

[103] The "vigorous" one, not the "lazy pumping" one.

Occasional ED is not a medical condition. Occasional ED will happen eventually to all guys one day or another. The causes are usually temporary (see below) and limited in time and generally do not require any medical assistance. Although an occasional ED can be really embarrassing vis-à-vis your partner in bed (or wherever), there is usually no need for worry except if this induces a state of regular anxiety which can than lead to a permanent ED.

Real erectile dysfunctions are those that require medical assistance. They are those were the penis remains totally limb and looks like an overcooked spaghetti. If this occurs on a regular basis, medical assistance is required. Soft erections should not be taken lightly as they can be due to chronic causes (which may require medical help) or occasional causes (usually they do not require medical help).

Here is a short (non exhaustive) list of causes of erectile dysfunction.

19.2.1. Psychological causes

These causes include stress, performance anxiety, fatigue, negative feelings, depression, etc. It is well known that stress, anxiety or fatigue are the main (and most common) reasons for not being able to get a good erection. To the contrary erections are usually strong in the morning when one is feeling relaxed. Unsurprisingly psychological illnesses or conditions can lead to ED.

So if you are tired and not able to pull up a boner, or if you are totally stressed at banging an incredibly hot/attractive girl (or guy) and not able to get hard, don't worry as this is this is just due to fatigue/anxiety.

If you tend to be depressed or have other psychological issues, consult a medical doctor if you have ED. If you take certain medicines, it becomes even more important to seek medical help.

19.2.2. Medical causes

There are many illnesses which can affect the blood flow or the nervous systems. These conditions may lead to ED and require medical help. Here are some of the well known cases:

- Prostate cancer/ prostate surgery/ lower abdomen surgery: sometimes the removal of anatomical structures can lead to nerve damage or an impaired supply of blood which can lead to ED even though the prostate itself is not required for an erection.

- Kidney failure, multiple sclerosis, diabetes: they can cause issues with blood supply and with the nervous systems.

- Disorders with the penis itself: neurological disorders, medical conditions of the corpus cavernosum.

19.2.3. Natural causes

Aging is a natural cause for ED (either full ED or soft erections) as the blood flow becomes gradually impaired through atherosclerosis. In some rare cases the decrease of testosterone can lead to ED. In this case a hormone replacement therapy may be required. However this can only be decided by a medical doctor. Do not start such therapies on your own as they can lead to severe problems including ED! More on testosterone is written in chapter 19.4 below.

19.2.4. Lifestyle causes

Like so many things, our lifestyle also can impact our erections. Obesity or just being overweight increases the risk of atherosclerosis which reduces the blood flow everywhere in the body, including in the penis. Diabetes just makes things worse.

Smoking also affects negatively erections due to its vasoconstrictor factors which will narrow arteries and therefore the blood supply to the corpus cavernosum.

19.2.5. Other causes

Another cause of "soft erections" is the one known as "porn addiction". Indeed, it has been established that those looking at too much porn for too long eventually respond less and less well to a "normal" level of stimuli which means in plain English that they can fap like monkeys in front of the PC but are less capable of erections with a real life partner. This is accentuated if they tend to masturbate with a "too tight" grip that is far from the sensation of a real body.

For the same reason, excessive masturbation can lead to soft erections.

These causes tend not to be permanent. Once the primary cause is removed (i.e. when you reduce the time spent looking at porn), things return should return to normal.

19.3. Ten tips to improve your erections

There are several factors that help increase the strength of erections.

1. Eat healthy (avoid junk foods). As said before, saturated fats tend to reduce the production of testosterone and increase the relative production of estrogens in men.

2. Use it or lose it as goes the saying. If you don't have regular intercourse (or masturbate) you will eventually get weaker erections.

3. Avoid smoking (due to consequences of vasoconstriction and lower blood supply to the penis).

4. Avoid alcohol (due to its impact on testosterone production).

5. Avoid excessive masturbation which can decrease your sexual appetite. You should try to save most of your energy for Mr. or Mrs. Right, not for Mr. Five Fingers.

6. Know the right positions! Warm up with oral sex to get the blood flowing. At the beginning use sexual positions like the missionary and doggy style which allow more blood to flow leading to a stronger and harder erection. To the contrary don't let your partner ride you first: the law of gravity is not your friend in this case[104].

7. Avoid tight undergarments. Avoid tight pyjamas which can restrict blood flow to penile tissues. Just sleep naked, it's easier.

8. Stay calm, avoid any anxiety factors. Nothing keeps a dick in "spaghetti mode" as well as anxiety or stress[105].

---

[104] This is why in porn movies the pros use most of the time the same sequence: oral, then missionary/doggy and only after "riding". At least, that is what I was told...

[105] If your partner is stressed or anxious, it's therefore important for you to realize this and then start by focusing on making him feel relaxed.

9. Exercise. This will improve your blood flow. In addition to traditional physical exercises, you can give your pelvic muscles a workout though Kegel exercises (like for women). Strengthening the pelvic muscles has shown the following benefits for men:

- reducing risk of incontinence,
- strengthening erections,
- reducing risk of premature ejaculation.

Men can follow the same Kegel routine as the one mentioned above for women, i.e.:

   a. Contract the pelvic muscles for 5-8 seconds, then relax for 5 seconds (this is one repetition),

   b. Do 10-15 repetitions before taking a 2 minute break (this is called one series),

   c. Do a total of 3-4 series every two or three times per week.

10. Make sure you get enough zinc in your food (zinc is involved in the synthesis of testosterone).

As said before, do consult a medical doctor if you have ED problems, especially if you take medicines on a regular basis for other medical conditions. Do note also that all the ads you see on the internet to make your penis longer or get stronger erections are just bogus. And the plastic tube gadgets where you put in your penis before pumping out the air in order to get a bigger dick are bogus at the best, but can be dangerous. You have been warned!

19.4. A few words on testosterone

Testosterone in men is essentially produced in the testicles and is responsible for the development of the male sexual characteristics. Testosterone is also important for maintaining muscle bulk, adequate levels of red cells, bone growth and sexual function.

As a man ages, his testosterone production will gradually decline after he is 25-30 years old. By itself the decline in testosterone is not, in most cases, the cause for ED.

Other factors can affect negatively testosterone production, including:

- Injury, infection or loss of the testicles,
- Chemotherapy,
- Dysfunctions of the pituitary gland (a gland in the brain which is responsible for the production of certain hormones),
- Certain medications (corticosteroids, etc),
- Chronic illnesses,
- Chronic kidney failure,
- Liver cirrhosis,
- Obesity.

Low testosterone can lead to the following conditions:

- Decrease in muscle mass with an increase in body fat,
- Changes in cholesterol levels,
- Osteoporosis[106],
- Decrease in body hair.

As said above, only a medical doctor can determine (after one or several blood tests) that a man has a condition known as "low testosterone". In this case a testosterone replacement therapy will be prescribed and the testosterone will given through intramuscular injections, patches on the skin, gel, oral tablets or subcutaneous implants.

---

[106] Indeed, osteoporosis can also be seen in men.

Testosterone replacement therapy should not be done if there is a case of prostate cancer or breast cancer[107].

Of course, like with any hormone replacement therapy, a medical follow-up is required. Indeed there can be side-effects with testosterone replacement therapy including:

- Acne,
- Worsening of sleep apnea,
- Decreased testicular size (since the body "realizes" that it no longer needs to produce as much testosterone),
- Increased aggression and mood swings,
- Changes in cholesterol levels,
- Decrease in sperm count and increased infertility (especially in younger men).

19.5. A few words on the sex pills to treat erectile dysfunction

Since Viagra, several sex pills have come out, including Cialis, Levitra and others. While many fake and counterfeit versions exist on the internet, the actual medicines have proven to be quite positive. The molecules in these pills are PDE5 inhibitors. Wow! That really does make me look smart! PDE5 inhibitors are molecules which will basically block signals to the smooth muscle cells lining the blood vessels supplying the corpus cavernosum of the penis. Basically, PDE5 inhibitors will block the signals which would lead the muscle cells of the arteries to contract and to reduce the blood supply to the corpus cavernosum.

Unlike what some people believe, these sex pills are not going to lead to having an erection right away or to get a boner at any point in time. Stimulation is necessary. However with the right stimuli, the boners become quite difficult to hide and go away. Since it's advised

---

[107] Although this is rare, men can also develop breast cancer as they also do have some breast tissue.

that the pills be taken 1-2 hours before planned intercourse, avoid any potentially embarrassing set-ups like having to do a presentation in front of people...

Such drugs are potent and can lead to adverse side effects such as head aches, loss of peripheral vision, priapism, heart attacks, increased intraocular pressure, sudden hearing loss, etc. This is why such drugs should be prescribed to you by a medical doctor only. Any side effect should lead you to stop taking these pills immediately and consult with your medical doctor.

19.5.1. Other facts on the sex pills

Many men, even those without ED, have started using these pills for recreational use. Recently a guy was telling me how, during his summer vacations in Asia, he took several of these pills and then went out to bang three hookers at the same time until he basically "wore them out" and "exhausted them" two and a half hours later. He added to me that he could have continued even longer but that he was hungry and "fed up". Many guys do this kind of stuff. However, and as said above, there can be side effects to these sex pills. There have been several cases related by the media where young men died of heart attacks after gobbling up too many pills in an effort to "please" their "numerous" partners.

On another subject, some scientists found that Viagra helps jet lag recovery in hamsters (no tests done on humans yet), while others found that putting dissolved Viagra in a vase of water can increase the shelf life of cut flowers... I wonder from where they got the funding for such research projects. Seems like being a scientist can be quite fun after all...

19.6. A few words on the use of anabolic steroids and other substances

In certain sports, there is a wide spread use of anabolic steroids, as well as other substances including testosterone, human growth hormone and insulin in order to increase muscle mass and muscle strength. These practices are dangerous and can lead to many serious, life threatening conditions including cardiovascular diseases, kidney failure, liver failure, breathing shortness and other respiratory problems, acne and skin problems, unwanted bone growth (especially jaw), increase in visceral fat just to name a few. Erectile dysfunction is another frequent side effect. Indeed, since the body "realizes" that it gets testosterone without doing anything, it will stop producing it itself. This leads to testicles which become as small as raisins (no joke). This often leads to erectile dysfunction.

Another problem is that if the testicles remain "inactive" for long enough, this can lead to hormonal imbalances which may require long term treatments though hormone replacement therapy. Bottom line: stay "natural" and avoid anabolic steroids and other substances to gain muscle strength and mass. You will gain less muscle, but you will not be putting your health at risk. It is well documented that many professional bodybuilders have sustained serious medical conditions during or after their career. The body has a memory. Sooner or later, it will remind you of the excesses you made.

19.7. Male baldness

Adults tend to have in between 100'000 and 150'000 hairs and lose an average of 100 hairs on a daily basis. If the losses of hair exceed the new hair, baldness appears. Male baldness (hereafter baldness) is above all a genetic factor. If you're a guy, there is a 4 out of 7 chance that you got the baldness gene, i.e. a 57% chance. Approximately 25% of men experience some form of hair loss before age 30, and 66% by age 60.

The trigger for baldness is DHT (dihydrotestosterone) which is an androgen (hormone that controls the development of the male characteristics). DHT is produced from testosterone after a chemical reaction (approx. 5% of testosterone gets transformed into DHT in the prostate). DHT is very important in the development of the embryo during pregnancy as it has an essential role in the development of the male external genitalia. For adults, DHT has mainly an impact on the brain (male character), libido, and the hair follicles (if you have the baldness gene) which brings us back to baldness. Indeed DHT will lead to a miniaturization of the hair follicle which will eventually deteriorate.

19.7.1. Other causes of baldness

While the genetic factor is by far the most important, there are other factors than cause hair thinning or hair loss:

- Traction: ponytails that pull the hair with excessive force tend to damage the cuticle (the outer casing of the hair) thus leading to damaged hair. Rigorous brushing can reinforce the problem.

- Medications such as those to treat high blood pressure, diabetes and cholesterol can lead to a temporary or permanent hair loss. Generally speaking, any kind of medication that impacts the body's hormonal balance can lead to hair loss. Anabolic steroids are an example of such drugs.

- Poor nutrition: deficiencies of protein, zinc, iron, vitamin B can cause hair thinning. While hair thinning is not baldness, it is often an aggravating factor. Diets with high animal fats (often found in fast foods) also are thought to have an impact on hair loss.

- Air and water pollutants, together with the effects of the sunlight, can also cause hair thinning by aging the scalp and damaging hair. Generally anything that can lead to damage of the scalp is a risk factor for hair. Some of the chemicals in certain shampoos/hair lotions may make the hair shine but are not necessarily good for the scalp (e.g. synthetic emulsifiers and detergents).

- Radiation (chemotherapy, Fukushima).

- Stress. Excessive levels of a stress related hormone (corticotrophin releasing hormone) will lead to hair loss.

A few words on remedies against baldness: they don't exist. Let me repeat: there are no remedies against baldness. None. Nada. Get over it, stop whining, live with it and suck it up. There are some authorized medicines that help slow the hair loss process, but they really don't have any significant impact over time. Some guys go on to wear wigs, others get into hair transplant (which is a really painful procedure).

A good looking bald guy will always look better than a hairy potato couch. Remember Kojak? Remember Mr. Clean? Remember Bruce Willis or Samuel L. Jackson to name a few? Today shaving the head has become totally sociably acceptable and even a sign of masculinity according to surveys. Therefore balding is really not an issue. So if you're balding, shave your head, go to the gym and you'll be doing just fine.

Chapter 20: Beauty tips

What? Beauty tips in a book about nutrition? You may think that I may have nothing to do tonight as I am writing. Maybe. Maybe not. The truth is that some of the big food companies have started to get into "neutraceuticals" which is the cross-road in between food, cosmetics and pharmaceuticals. The idea is that to look good from outside, you need to be healthy from inside. We have seen, for many years now, yogurts filled with active bifid bacterium used as probiotics[108] in order to improve the intestinal flora. In the same fashion, many of the multi-mineral/multi-vitamin pills contain minerals and vitamins which are used for many biological processes, which in some case involve "beauty".

As goes the saying: "beauty is in the eye of the beholder". Many women seem to find Daniel Craig the ultimate hot alpha male. I find him both skinny and fat. It seems that at the gym he only works out his pecs. Of course, each person has different tastes and each woman will have a different judgment on whether Daniel Craig is hot or not[109].

Anyways, here are a few lines on beauty tips for which nutrition is part of the solution.

20.1. Wrinkles

Wrinkles are a fold or a crease in the skin. They usually appear as the result of the aging process. Let's be frank: wrinkles do not look

---

[108] Probiotics are live bacteria which may confer health benefits on the host.

[109] Straight men are less complicated in their criteria for beauty. Indeed for most of them beauty can be summarized as "a pair of big boobs". On the other side, some of the gay men have a much more aesthetic view of beauty which is why many tend to really take care of themselves and the way they look. I don't want to seem to complain, but in my personal experience I can confirm that during my workouts at the gym, those that are looking at me are usually guys and not chicks. Sigh! :/

nice. They make you look much older than what you would otherwise look like. So here are some tricks to avoid (or at least reduce) the wrinkles you will eventually get:

1. Protect the skin from the sun:

Sun damages the skin in several ways. First it will dehydrate the skin which over times increases the wrinkles as the skin's ability to retain water becomes impaired. Second, the sun will increase the damage to genes. Genetic mutations in skin exposed to sun were found 2-3x higher than skin not exposed to sun. Since genes control the production and strength of collagen (which is the protein that confers elasticity to the skin), a higher number of mutations increases the probability of a decrease in collagen production as well as the production of a weaker collagen.

2. Drink a lot (all the time, not only in summer)

The more you hydrate your body, the more you hydrate your skin. Creams to hydrate the skin are nice and good. However, it's the water you drink that really hydrates the skin from the inside.

3. Consume a lot of anti-oxidants

I have mentioned in several places the importance of anti-oxidants as a means to reduce the damage of oxygen free radicals to DNA and other vital molecules. Anti-oxidants will help reduce the damages to your skin as well.

4. Wear sunglasses

Sunglasses protect the delicate skin around the eyes. They also help avoid squinting which directly contributes to the wrinkles around the eyes.

5. Avoid smoking

Smoke damages the collagen over time, therefore leading to increase wrinkles. Smokers tend to have many more wrinkles than non smokers. The vasoconstriction impact of some of the substances contained in the smoke will over time reduce the blood flow, especially to the smaller vessels which are near the skin. This will accelerate the aging process of the skin for smokers.

6. Avoid excessive facial expressions

In the face, the use of facial expressions is the main driver for wrinkles. Try to avoid excessive facial expressions.

7. Sleep enough

As mentioned in chapter 16.3., it's during sleep that most of the human growth hormone is produced and that your body gets repaired. Not enough sleep will favor wrinkles.

The skin is delicate, especially where there is less "meat" and where the risk of dehydration is the greatest. Unsurprisingly, the under-eyes are probably the most vulnerable area. If you smoke, if you take too much sun or don't sleep enough, the under-eyes will show it first. Unfortunately, unlike other areas of the body, the skin cannot be repaired. You hear this right, like atherosclerosis, like spinal disc damage and other things, it's simply not possible to repair skin damage. Sure you can put creams and other things to hide the problems, but they will not disappear. That's why it's critical to take care of your skin if you want to look young. Therefore, even in summer, stay cool! Stay in the shade! Drink a lot of water and go to bed early[110].

---

[110] Of course, only do this if you're not single. If you're single and do this, you will probably stay single for much longer than what you expected.

20.2. Saggy skin and breast ptosis

With age, skin can become saggy in certain areas. It's the effect of the gravity as well the effect of the progressive damage to the collagen which leads the skin to become distended.

For women, this problem is the most acute for their breasts, especially those that are heavier and that have sustained more damages from sun exposure, dehydration or smoking.

The medical term for saggy boobs is ptosis. Since breasts do not contain muscle, physical exercise cannot help. Breasts are not protected from external forces (gravity), and unlike what some women believe, bras do not prevent ptosis. Actually recent studies have shown that bras actually *increase* ptosis as the skin tissue does not need to "support itself" and "relies" on something else.

As said above, while some degree of ptosis is "normal", it can be reduced by taking some of the steps mentioned above in chapter 20.1., i.e.:

- Avoid excessive sun exposure on the breasts (especially those heaver ones),
- Hydrate properly,
- Sleep enough,
- Don't smoke,
- Try (when possible) not no wear bras (e.g. at home) where you can just use a t-shirt,
- Consume a lot of anti-oxidants and avoid taking too many saturated fatty acids.

Of course, plastic surgery can correct heavy cases of ptosis. But in most cases, following the tips indicated above should be enough to keep the breasts in shape.

In other areas of the body, where muscle is near, saggy skin can be reduced through physical exercise. Many women eventually tend to have saggy triceps (the under part of the arm for those not into anatomy). This can clearly be addressed by bodybuilding exercises.

So there is no excuse for saggy arms! Of course, bodybuilding for women will also help strengthen and tone the other body parts where fat may start to accumulate: often hips, booty, legs and abdomen. For men, the issue of saggy skin also exists, although to a lesser extent since the percentage of body fat is higher in women than in men and since the latter tend to have more muscle. Here too, if you're a guy and don't want to have your pecs touch your belly button, or if you don't want to have your belly skin hanging down, bodybuilding to strengthen your muscles is required. Cardio will help you lose weight, but to avoid having the "excessive" skin just "hanging" there, you will need to replace the fat you had by muscle.

Chapter 21: A few words on antioxidants

I have mentioned in numerous occasions the importance and role of antioxidants as a way to reduce the damage incurred by important biological molecules (in particular DNA) due to various oxygen containing molecules known as free radicals. Since these free radicals have an electric imbalance (lack or excess of electrons), they will seek to find an electric balance through the combination with another molecule. In order to avoid that this be done with important molecules such as DNA, these free radicals need to be neutralized by other molecules.

The body does produce antioxidants. Antioxidants can also be found in certain foods/drinks. In other cases, some of the elements needed to produce antioxidants within the body are found in certain foods/drinks. This is for the example of selenium and zinc which are required for the activity of certain antioxidant enzymes.

Before getting in on the details of antioxidants, I would like to write a few words on sports. Doing physical exercise by definition involves a bigger intake of oxygen than when you are relaxing, and thus intense sport efforts will generate a state of high level oxidation. This is why proper nutrition is critical when doing physical exercises. What you eat before, during and after exercising is key.

21.1. The main human antioxidants

Antioxidants can be water soluble or fat soluble (lipid soluble). Water soluble antioxidants will tend to react with the oxidants found in the blood and found in the liquid within the cell (cystol or intracellular fluid) whereas the lipid soluble antioxidants will react with the oxidant agents found in the cell membranes.

All of these antioxidants are essential against diseases such as cancer, but also other diseases which result from the degeneration of cells, including Alzheimer, Parkinson's or glaucoma to name a few.

Some of the main human soluble antioxidants are the following:

1. Ascorbic acid (vitamin C) – water soluble:

Vitamin C cannot be synthesized by the body but has to be ingested in the frame of the diet. Fruits are the main sources of vitamin C. Multi-mineral/multi-vitamin pills also include vitamin C.

2. Uric acid – water soluble:

This is the antioxidant which has the highest concentration in the blood. It is produced by enzymes in the frame of complex chemical reactions which are beyond the scope of this book.

3. Glutathione – water soluble

This is the antioxidant which has the highest concentration in the liver tissue. Here too, I will not dwell on its chemical production.

4. Vitamin E – lipid soluble

Vitamin E can be found in many vegetable oils, nuts, seeds and whole grains. Multi-mineral/multi-vitamin pills also include vitamin E.

5. Carotenes (beta carotene and retinol (vitamin A) – lipid soluble

These molecules can be found in sweet potatoes, carrots, spinach, beets, broccoli, parsley, pumpkin, etc.

6. Ubiquinol – lipid soluble

This molecule is produced through chemical reactions involving enzymes.

21.2. Other antioxidant molecules

There are other antioxidant molecules, not produced by the human body, which can also help reduce the degradation of vital molecules.

21.2.1. Phenols, polyphenols and flavonoids

Phenols and polyphenols are compounds found in plants. A sub group called the flavonoids is the one that research identified has having the highest potential to contribute to better health.

While medical research studies have sometimes been found contradictory, there is growing evidence that a nutrition based on the intake of higher proportions of these molecules helps reduce certain illnesses or health conditions.

Flavonoids can be found in citrus (lemons, grapefruits), berries, onions, red onions, parsley, green tea, red wine, dark chocolate among others.

Green tea has among the highest contents of flavonoids among food and beverages. Molecules like catechins, tannins and theaflavins are well known[111]. Rooibos (a.k.a. red tea) also contains high levels of aspalathin and nothofagin. It also contains other flavanols, flavones and dihydrochalcones[112] and is said to help with nervous tension, allergies and digestive problems.

Red wine contains tannins, as well as flavonols and anthocyanins.

---

[111] Okay, maybe the term "well known" is a bit of an overstatement and clearly the "bling bling" community in Los Angeles may not know them. However these are molecules you may read in health articles.
[112] I only included these names to help you next time you play scrabble.

Part 7: Further reading

You want to learn more on nutrition and physical exercises? You want to learn more about your truth? Congrats! That's the spirit!

Here are some references for further reading, as well as other places on internet that can be of interest.

Lose weight now!

Chapter 22: Further reading

This chapter will be short. But there is no need to really make it long after all.

All I want to say is that this book is only the first step in your new lifestyle. It is quite clear that you can apply the guidelines of this book. However you will have to adapt your nutrition and physical exercises to your age, gender and overall health condition. You will need to go through trial and error to fine tune what you do as far as nutrition and sports to what works the best for your body. Do remember that you are unique, and what may work for one person may not work for you.

There are tons of sources of information to help you. You can, and should, start with your medical doctor. Then of course, check out the internet of course. It's an unlimited, ever expanding source of information. Just be careful as you will find a lot of rubbish there, as well as conflicting views. However, it's by reading different opinions, analyzing them with your mind, and in some cases testing them, that you will find your own truth. But make no mistake, with all the free resources out there, your own research may put you on par with many medical doctors on certain topics.

I would like nevertheless like to mention one site which I found very informative about the nutritional composition of food. The breakdown of proteins, carbs, lipids and minerals is given. You also can see the detail of what kind of carbs, what kind of proteins (amino acids), what kind of lipids each food has. The link is below:

http://nutritiondata.self.com/facts/dairy-and-egg-products/118/2

Of course there are other similar sites which give many details of the foods and drinks we eat. The idea is nevertheless that while counting carbs and calories is really quite useless in my opinion[113], you should be aware of things like:

- How much protein does this food have?

- How much saturated fats does this food have?

- I'm looking to increase my intake of antioxidants. What should I consume?

- I am diabetic, what are the foods that don't have high levels of simple carbs?

- I need to increase my intake of dietary fibers to help my intestinal transit. What foods should I eat?

- I sometimes have heavy periods, what should I take to increase my iron intake?

---

[113] As said previously, what matters is the balance in between food intake (calories intake) and physical exercise (calories spent).

Conclusion

All good things come to an end, and so has this book[114]. But I need to finish first the conclusion. What should I write? Should I call someone else to help give me inspiration? I guess not. With the nice weather I'm quite sure everybody's chilling somewhere.

So how should I finish this book? I'm not going to summarize this book. No need for another ten pages.

Should I apologize to some of the producers of diet methods or diet gurus for criticizing their tools and techniques? Hell no! They need no compassion from my side. Anyways they will probably continue to prosper for ages and ages to come. Unfortunately human nature doesn't change, and the "easy way" will always attract many people in the future as it has over the past.

While I cannot change the fate of the many, I hope to modestly help some to decide to change their lives.

I will end this conclusion by telling the obvious truth.

All humans are products of the stars. The atoms of our bodies were created in the fusion reactions at the heart of stars and in supernovae reactions in some of the biggest stars in our galaxy.

We all have the ability, through our will and determination, to change our lives and try to inspire positively the ones of our relatives. The same why that unhealthy lifestyles are transmitted from parents to their children and so forth, a health lifestyle adopted by parents can then inspire the children and break the vicious circle of obesity, sedentary life and content with mediocrity.

---

[114] If you found this book totally annoying, rejoice! It's almost over! Yaaay!

Changing our lifestyle is not easy. It takes time and commitment. The path is not known in advance, and each one of us will have to draw his or her own road map. The route will often be filled with traps and obstacles put there to test our determination. We will sometimes get lost and go through detours. However we should keep the correct direction in mind and, despite the challenges, keep moving in the direction of our goals and dreams.

Life is not a destination, but a journey as goes the saying. So I will end up with a few lines from a song of an American music group from Chicago[115]:

> *You are your Master*
> *So set your soul free*
> *Forget your stupid idols*
> *And your blinded eyes will see*

Thanks again, Dear Reader, for taking the time to read my book. I hope that, in one way or another, it will help you on your path to achieving some of your personal goals.

Again, thanks for reading, and keep looking up!

Peace,

Antonio
May 25, 2015

www.loseweight.ch
info@loseweight.ch

---

[115] The group is called « Master » and the lyrics are from their self-titled song.

Antonio Macerata

Lose weight now!

If you are reading these lines, you have either not realized that the book is over, or you have started by the wrong side.